S0-AKW-984

Vintage Fashions for Women

The 1950s & 60s

Kristina Harris

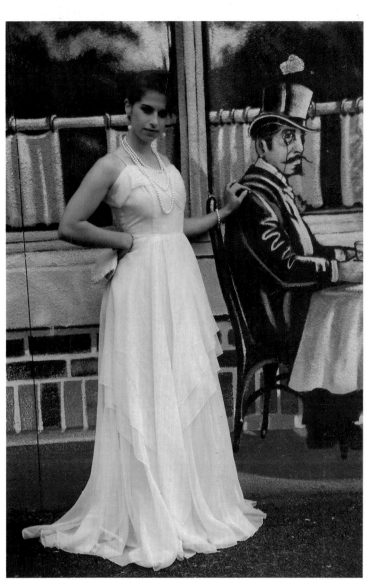

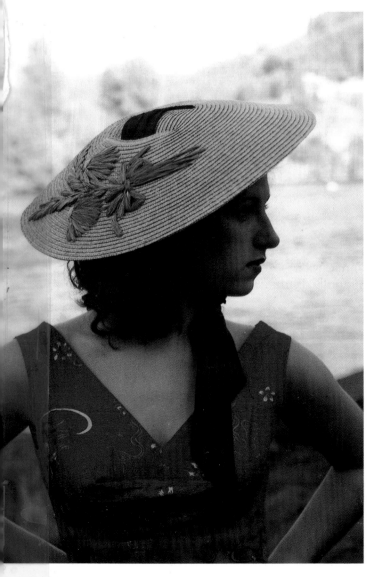

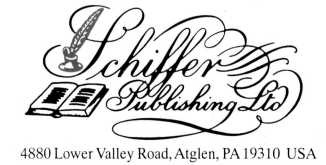

4880 Lower Valley Road, Atglen, PA 19310 USA

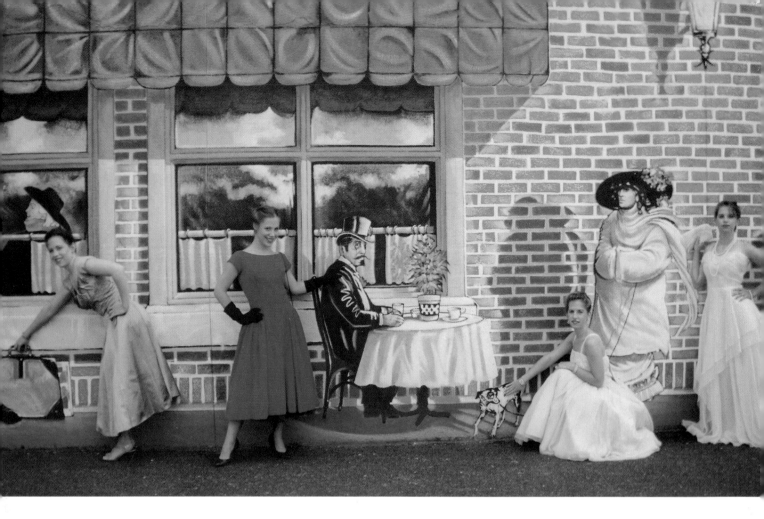

The styles of the 1950s and early 1960s echoed Victorian
fashions.

Copyright © 1997 by Kristina Harris

All rights reserved. No part of this work may be reproduced or
used in any form or by any means—graphic, electronic, or
mechanical, including photocopying or information storage
and retrieval systems—without written permission from the
copyright holder.

Designed by "Sue"

ISBN: 0-7643-0197-7
Printed in Hong Kong

Published by Schiffer Publishing Ltd.
4880 Lower Valley Road
Atglen, PA 19310
Phone: (610) 593-1777; Fax: (610) 593-2002
Please write for a free catalog.
This book may be purchased from the publisher.
Please include $2.95 for shipping.
Try your bookstore first.

We are interested in hearing from authors
with book ideas on related subjects.

Library of Congress Cataloging-in--Publication Data

Harris, Kristina.
    Vintage fashions for women: the 1950s and 60s
Kristina Harris.
        p. cm.
    Includes index.
    ISBN 0-7643-0197-7 (paper)
    1.Costume--United States--History--20th century.
2. Vintage clothing--United States. 3. Costume--United
States--History--20th century--Collectors and collecting.
I. Title.
GT615.H373   1997
391' .2'097309045--dc21   97-6979
                                               CIP

Title page, bottom left photo:
Many designs were inspired by Mexican
and Oriental motifs.

Top right photo:
The wide variety of styles—from sophisticated to youthful—make the era of the
1950s-60s especially rich for collectors.

Contents

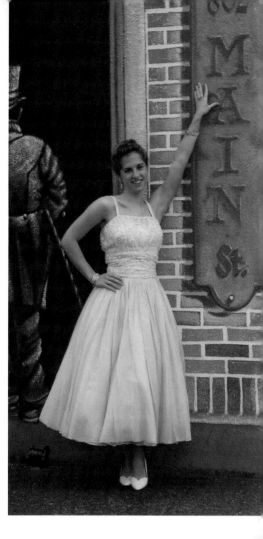

Chiffon was a fabric of choice in evening wear.

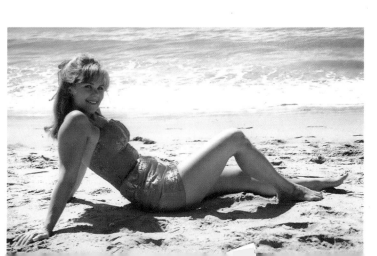

Bathing suits most often covered the body modestly, but were strikingly attractive.

Acknowledgments

This book wouldn't have been nearly as much fun to create—nor offer even half its brio—if it weren't for the models. Each devoted time and energy generously. I am especially grateful to Anna Kristine Crivello, Clinton McKay Crivello, Lisa Ann Crivello, Joslin Gordon, Darcie Jones, and Stephanie Jones—all of whom have been a steady part of not only this book, but also *Victorian & Edwardian Fashions for Women: 1840-1919* and *Vintage Fashions For Women: 1920s-1940s*. Newcomers Jennifer Yarascak and Lisa Dunn also deserve warm thanks. For smiling and looking beautiful (or handsome!) on chilly, rainy days, and hot, sticky days, being poked by safety pins, and so much more—thank you all.

Thank you, thank you to my mother and her museum O.F.C., and old and new friends Diane Seldman, Jerry Bickmore, D. Lisa Rand, and Bill Dauphin for lending pieces from their collections. I also thank The Very Little Theatre in Eugene, Oregon, for once again allowing me access to their antique and vintage clothing collection; Lucy Sullivan deserves great blessings for all her work at V.L.T.—including the enthusiasm and time she offered me during this project. As always, Lucy, your participation is greatly appreciated. Thanks also to Mary Mason for background information on her lovely duds; the enthusiasm you always overflow with is inspiring, dah-ling!

Particular thanks also goes to Sue Gustafson of Flossy McGrew's vintage clothing in Denver, Colorado, who not only responded enthusiastically to my query for paper dresses, but also got caught up in the excitement of this project and lent a myriad of other wonderful fashions. In addition, Rosetta Hurley of Persona Vintage Clothing in Astoria, Oregon, was kind as always and lent generously—as did Marlene Minnich of Marianie's Vintage Chic in Lehighton, Pennsylvania. For sharing their paper dresses, I also thank Karla Luallen of Klassic Line Vintage Clothing in Wichita, Kansas and Rose Ogden of Annie's Antique Mall, also in Wichita.

Though many of the photographs in this book were taken with our beautiful Oregon nature as a backdrop, many people and organizations also kindly offered wonderful man-made sites and props. My thanks are extended to: Jan Alberg of The Shelton-McMurphy-Johnson House in Eugene, Oregon; mural artist Pat Curtis (and the City of Springfield, Oregon for all their wonderful murals); The Lively Park Swim Center, also in Springfield, Oregon; the Beach Boardwalk in Santa Cruz, California; and James Conn for his delightful 1957 Corvette.

Last, but by no means least, I thank my father, Jerry Harris, for allowing me to photograph in his lovely garden (and for supporting my fashion-collecting habit by donating a number of beautiful garments), and my mother, Gretchen Harris, who offered a legion of support services—from helping me gather and haul clothing, to lending an extra pair of hands while digging through piles of period magazines at antique shops, to offering her expert advice on the clothes of "her" era.

And no acknowledgment is truly complete without thanking all of you who have read my books and written wonderful letters to me; you are a special bunch, and you inspire me.

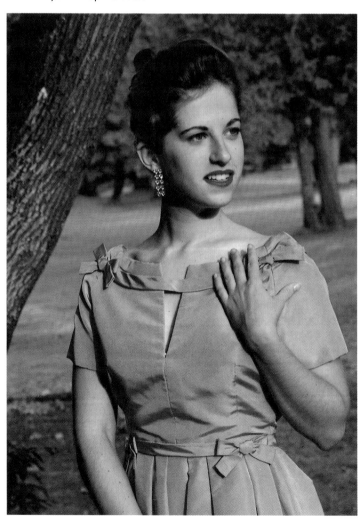

Couture designer Christian Dior shaped the fashions of the 1950s and early 60s.

Introduction

My first contact with the fashions of the 1950s-60s came when I was about 12 or 13 years old. While doing the usual teenage shopping for records (no CDs then) and costume jewelry, I came across a thrift store packed full of used clothing and accessories. I was stunned and delighted all at once. Stunned I hadn't discovered the store before, that *everyone* didn't shop there, and that there weren't a dozen of them in town. And delighted by the clothing which I deemed far more interesting and beautiful than anything I could buy at a department store—and much less expensive, besides. What a marvelous invention this "old clothes" shop was!

Soon, I had a small wardrobe of vintage fashions from this little shop—mostly fashions from the 1950s and early 1960s which I purchased to wear. I had no idea in those days—though my parents were ardent antique collectors and my mother an antiques dealer—that people actually collected clothing like they did old china or glassware. I remember particularly purchasing a black lace dress from the 1950s. At the time, I thought it very grown-up and even glamorous, though today I look back and think it was more youthful than I realized. With a full skirt supported by several layers of stiffened net, and a squared neckline trimmed with velvet and what I thought were the most enticing pom-poms, I wore the dress with great pride whenever I wanted to appear impressive. I was so taken with the dress, in fact, that I saved it, and it resides in my collection even today.

There were others, of course. A flirty, box-pleated knee-length skirt from the sixties, another lace dress—this one red—from the fifties, a Grace Kelly inspired long formal dress of faint green embellished with iridescent sequins, a purse composed of black beaded tassels from the sixties...the list grew every year, as did compliments on my manner of dress.

Today, teenagers still find "cheap chic" in the fashions of the fifties and sixties, but collectors—who once shunned such young fashions—now are also taking interest in the styles of this era. Unfortunately, very little has been written about the fashions of this period that is helpful to the collector. To remedy this was half my reason for writing this book. (The other half? To glory in those full-skirted or pencil-slim fashions as I did as a teenager!)

One of the chief problems in creating a collector's book on the fashions of the 1950s-60s is that there is such an abundance of it. Mass-marketing reached a pinnacle in the 1950s, and the number of manufacturers of women's clothing was astounding. Often, fashion magazines contradicted each other about which styles were most fashionable, and when new looks were introduced—unlike many 19th and early 20th century fashions—women didn't always gobble them up, believing that designers alone dictated fashions.

However, upon reviewing hundreds of copies of old magazines—primarily the middle-class variety like *Mademoiselle* and *Glamour* (not to mention sewing pattern magazines)—certain trends become clear. Sometimes, however, a fashion that would appear from the magazines to be widely popular, generating numerous ads from several manufacturers, is of a style that can rarely be found in today's marketplace. The photographs in this book, then, serve as a general guide to availability.

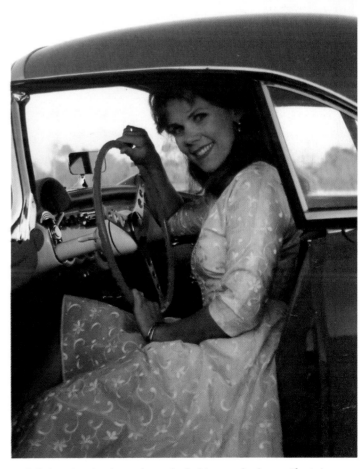

Reliving simpler times through clothing and other artifacts is one of the fastest-growing areas of American interest.

For many of the same reasons, readers will find that few of the garments photographed here are dated to a specific year. The ultimate reason for this is that fashions overlap so much. If you find this difficult to believe, try this little experiment: Study several modern fashion magazines (*Vogue* is a good example); now study what people in the streets are wearing. You'll find they most often wear clothing that was shown in fashion magazines a year—even five years—earlier.

As a collector, I have always been frustrated that most books focus only on couture designers—Chanel, Dior, and the rest of that elite gang. The vast majority of clothes were not created by these artists—yet they were designed by *someone*. Popular opinion has it that all new styles are invented by coutures, then copied by designers in the mass-marketing industry; however, the opposite may have, at least at times, been true. No one will ever really know, of course, because fashion magazines only report on couture designers' new collections—despite the fact that design ideas come from a variety of sources *outside* of the couture house. Up until the 1920s, this was often a dressmaker, seamstress, or home-sewer, but by the 1930s, it was most frequently designers whose fashions were distributed by mass-manufacturers. More than any earlier period, the 1950s-60s was the era of this latter sort of designer. And so, I have attempted to help these unsung heroes of fashion become recognized and appreciated. Though I couldn't hope to list all the many thousands of said designers producing in this era, I have focused on those who were most popular.

The fashions of the 1950s-60s are really for the thoughtful collector. Reason tells us that while these vintage fashions are still relatively "new," they will within decades be considered extremely collectible and be valued at least twice their worth today. By collecting today, however, the collector can choose from the best of the crop—and can do so even on a budget.

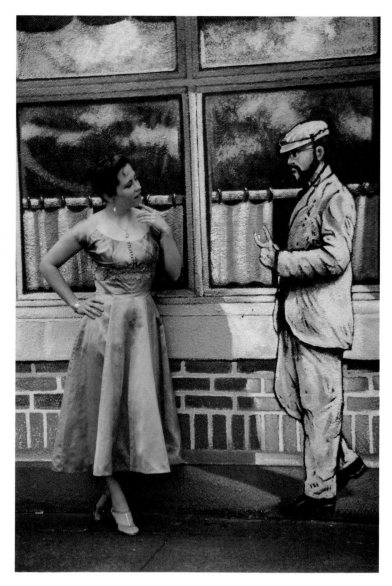

Many styles remained much the same in the sixties as they'd been in the fifties, but were frequently simplified and less fussy. *Courtesy of The Very Little Theatre.*

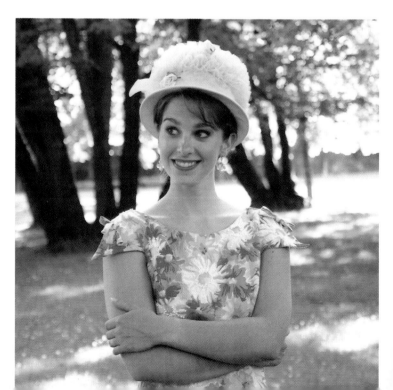

As the sixties progressed, the trend toward playful clothing only increased.

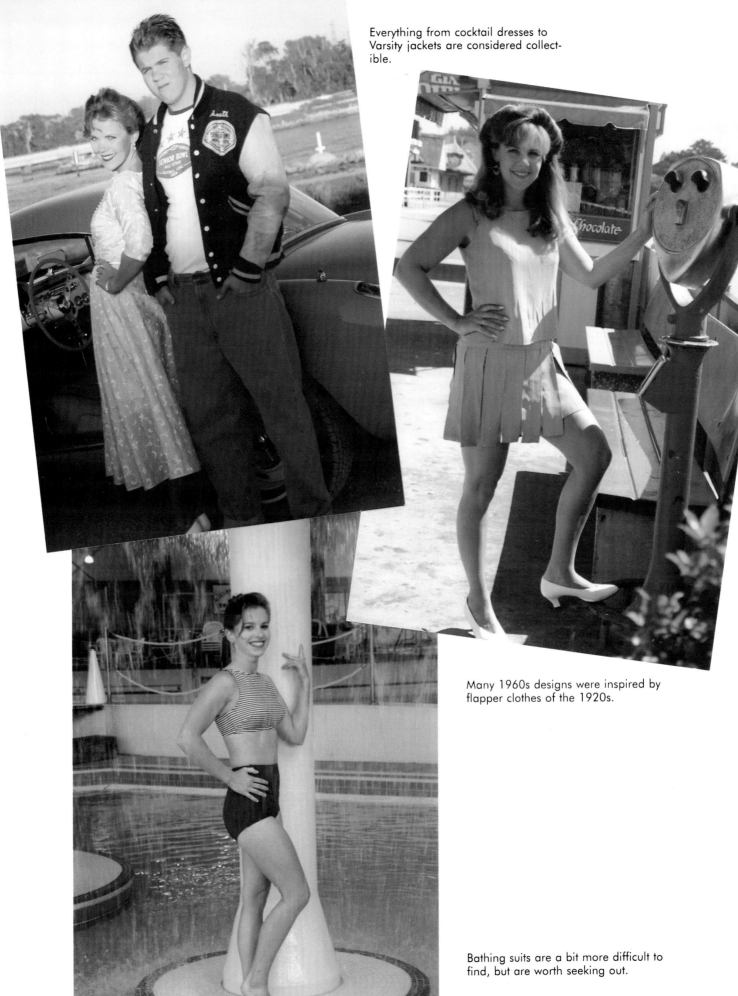

Everything from cocktail dresses to Varsity jackets are considered collectible.

Many 1960s designs were inspired by flapper clothes of the 1920s.

Bathing suits are a bit more difficult to find, but are worth seeking out.

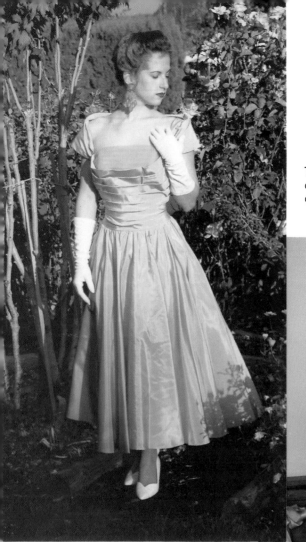

Teenage prom dresses are widely available to collectors and can be anything from wild to ultra-romantic.

There are many more excellent condition garments available from the 1950s on than from any earlier era.

Many fifties and early sixties formal gowns went after the Grace Kelly look.

PART ONE

You'll have to excuse me. I happen to have a passion for the fashions of the 1950s. Perhaps its because they embody all the important elements of Victorian fashions (another one of my passions)—but somehow seem more accessible, more down to earth. This is, after all, the concept that Christian Dior—the couture designer responsible for the look of the 1950s—had in mind when he first introduced postwar women to his sweeping skirts and fitted bodices.

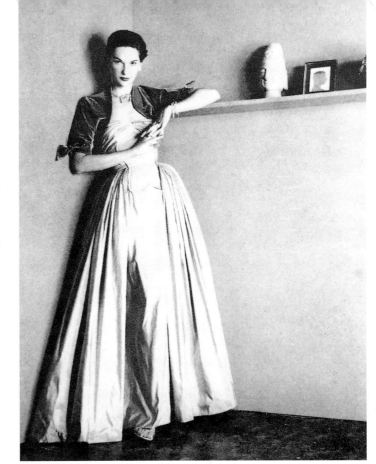

A 1952 Henri Bendel ad featuring a "New Look" evening gown of silk taffeta and silk velvet in emerald green for $295.

The 1950s

The "New" Old Look

Actually, this idea of neo-Victorian fashions was nothing new. In 1939, the couture designer known as Mainbocher (his real name was Main Rousseau Bocher), followed by a number of other designers, showed dresses in top fashion magazines like *Vogue* and *Harper's Bazaar* that featured ultra-curves and neo-Victorian motifs. But when the Second World War hit, women were anything but in the spirit to go backwards into fashion history. Instead adopting simplified styles that were both practical and met with war rationing restrictions, by the end of the war, women were starved for something new—something that would sweep them off their feet and refresh them after the devastations of world war. "You have a chance that seldom comes more than once in a lifetime," British *Vogue* wrote in July of 1945, "the chance to buy a completely new wardrobe." Christian Dior cleverly met that need.

"I wanted my dresses to be constructed, molded upon the curves of the feminine body, whose sweep they would stylize," Dior himself said. Launched in the spring of 1947, Dior called his refreshing new line *"corolle,"* the botanical term for the frail petals at the center of a flower. Fashion magazines immediately picked up on the fact that this new line was very much influenced by the designer's mother's lush Victorian fashions. "From the era of Madame Bovary," *Vogue* rhapsodized, "wasp-waisted Gibson Girl shirtwaists, pleated or tucked...slow-sloped, easy shoulders...wrapped and bound middles—barrel (almost hobble) skirts—longer, deeply shaped shadowbox décolleté—padded hips..." Soon, fashion magazines had re-dubbed Dior's line, giving it the name that struck a chord with women everywhere: "The New Look."

"I thought I had never seen such wonderful young women with their towering Marie Antoinette hairdos, topped with artificial flowers, plump with healthy porcelain complexions, with high pointed bosoms and 'cuisses' [corsets]. In fashionable restaurants the women were wearing, on their heads, enormous platters strewn with ostrich plumes or roses. It was as if the war had never been!" film costumer Cecil Beaton exclaimed upon visiting the United States.

As mass-manufacturers began imitating Christian Dior's "New Look" line, a new lady-like charm was being adopted by post-war women. "The New Look" took women back to the more simple, traditional days of their great-grandmothers, with fashions that were unquestionably feminine. "The New Look" transformed the square, padded shoulders of the war era into softer, more sloping shoulders. Boxy skirts metamorphosed and began curving inward toward the body or standing away from the legs in a bell shape reminiscent of the fashions worn by Mary Todd Lincoln. Dior suits were lightly padded along the hipline, or had flounces or peplums to give an exaggerated hour-glass figure to their wearer. Not since the turn of the century had the "wasp-figure" been so sought after by American women.

Separate bustles and hip pads could also be worn—purchased from manufacturers or made at home with a sewing pattern. Like their Victorian counterparts, these were comprised of either stiffened taffeta or silk, or of fabric stuffed and tied around the waist. Crinolines—another article stolen directly from the Victorians—were also revived. At first, plastic hoop-skirt style crinolines were favored, but worn with shorter skirts than had been worn in the 1800s, these had a tendency to tip up and reveal more than most women wished to expose. Dior preferred petticoats made of stiffened nylon; with a wide hip yolk and several layers of ruffled net plunging toward the floor, these crinolines became one of the signatures of the decade.

True Dior designs were also marked by incredible built-in support—making Dior's designs nearly stand up by themselves. Skirts were interlined with stiffened muslin and lined with taffeta or acetate. Hems were also lined with stiffened muslin or calico (usually brightly colored in case a flip of the skirt revealed the lining). And Pellon (a new-fangled stiffening fabric which could be ironed and stick directly onto the overfabric) often shaped entire skirts, holding them away from the legs in the new bell shape.

When Dior's "New Look" skirts were not full, they were nearly skin-tight. This made it necessary to line them with acetate and muslin to help stiffen and support the outer fabric, plus ward off "seating." Mass-produced skirts rarely had such good linings, but many women wore straight, firm underslips to achieve the same look.

Another essential ingredient of "The New Look" was the revival of the Victorian-style corset. Though women (whether they were plump or slim) had been wearing firm rubberized girdles for some forty years, Dior made the cinched-up corset seem like the newest thing—when in fact it was the oldest thing. Fashion magazines weren't eager to dub the contraption

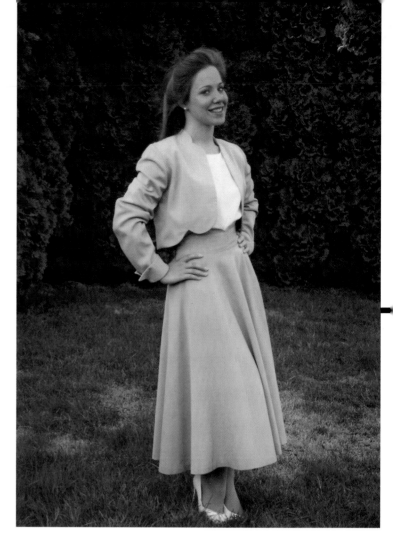

A home-made "New Look" suit. Though it still features some typical 1940s features (including thick shoulder pads) its softer lines and feminine scalloping epitomizes the years 1949-50. *Courtesy of Flossy McGrew's.*

a "corset," however (only three decades earlier, after all, they had made it their mission to murder the corset by giving it a bad name), and preferred creating more exotic terms for it, including "guêpière." Dior dubbed his own corset (which was famous for taking inches off the waistline) the "waspie." This modernized version of the Victorian corset was about five or six inches deep, made of ridged fabric with elastic inserts, and contained boning and back-lacing.

In addition to corsets, Dior often inserted feather boning into the waists of his skirts and dresses. For women who could only afford to buy the mass-produced version of "The New Look," *Vogue* suggested the use of a "waist-liner," which was apparently a strip of muslin or seam binding with boning sewn onto it, which *Vogue* said gave "a thin strip of indentation about [the] waist, and could be sewn into each...dress."

Yet not everyone sang Dior's praises. In early 1947 when Dior's line was first being introduced, war-devastated Europe experienced some of the coldest weather ever; fuel was in short supply; people were

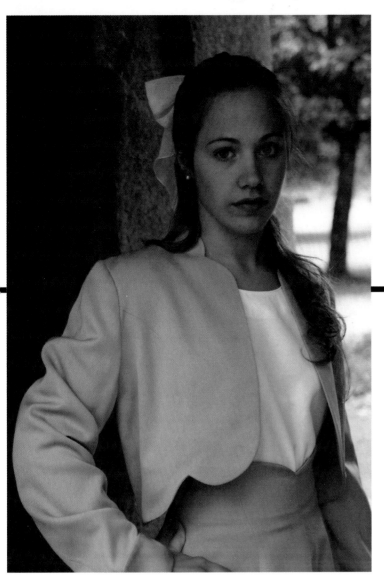

reaching to the ankle. Worn beneath this was a multi-layered stiff petticoat, attached with hooks and eyes to a sturdy waist yolk. The regale suit weighed nearly five pounds.

Yet by and large, Dior was beloved and his designs embraced by women rich and poor, young and old. "The New Look" became a hot catch-phrase, one that was added to numerous ad campaigns to help sell everything from pillows to tampons. And while actual Dior "New Look" designs didn't last much past 1950, every dress, every skirt or blouse, every hat, every glove of the 1950s and early 1960s was based upon Christian Dior's original "New Look" designs.

The Ready-To-Wear Boom

The 1950s were America's last "age of innocence." Women—though many had careers in addition to home lives—were supposed to be traditional "women," and men, bless them, were seen as "real men"—à la Grace Kelly and Kirk Douglas. The clothes of the era reflect these ideals. Every "smart" woman accessorized properly, marking herself as a lady by her choice of gloves, hat, shoes, bag, and jewelry. Henry Fairlie, writing for *Vogue*, commented that women had been hoodwinked. Despite the emancipation they'd received since the turn of the century, he claimed that women were now re-enslaved by their typewriters, and that make-up, fashion, and fashion magazines were "drugs to keep the slaves quiet." Nonetheless, many women felt they were achieving the best of both worlds—at least the best the 1950s could offer.

Though more concealing than fashions had been since the 1910s, the clothing of the 1950s weren't necessarily confining. Instead of revealing all, women were learning that it could be to their benefit to tempt the imagination with what was cleverly concealed. This, in fact, was the common theme in fifties clothing. Between a decade when many women hid under tailored suits and boxy dresses, and an era when half the population began favoring near-nudity, women of the fifties romanced the world with clothes that exposed little, but emphasized all.

But not all changes were taking place on the designer's sketch pad or in the consumer's mind. Mass-manufacturing, first begun in full force in the 1920s, was reaching an all-time pinnacle of achievement. Keeping up in a decade of affluence and commercialism (where having a TV antenna was important even if you couldn't actually afford a TV), mass-

dying from exposure; rationing and shortages were severe; and many were outraged by Dior's extravagant styles. At one point, when Dior's models were standing outside, waiting to do a photo shoot clothed in his latest designs, they were viciously attacked, their clothing nearly torn off them by women who were waiting nearby in long food lines.

And then there were those who saw "The New Look" as a set-back for women—a sign that women (who had finally begun to find success in the workforce) were suddenly being cast back into their Victorian role of housewife now that the war was over and their labor was no longer needed in order to preserve the economy. Though this may have been a symbolic interpretation of the new line, there were actual physical ramifications, as well. Take Dior's 1947 "Bar Suit," for example: a waist-nipping, long sleeved, high neckline jacket with a wide, stiffened, padded, and weighted peplum. The bell-shaped skirt required nearly six yards of fabric to create, featured sixty tight pleats, and measured eight yards around the hem,

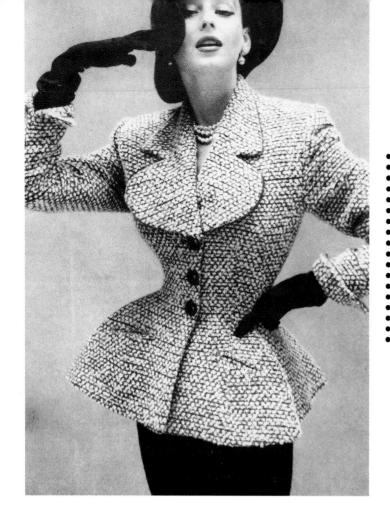

A "luxurious poodle cloth" jacket by Lilli Ann but showing extreme influence by Christian Dior designs.

"Q: 'Dear Ladies Home Journal:...Where, oh, where dear L.H.J., do you find all those beautiful girls for your covers and ads?' A: 'We have a peripatetic editor who goes all over the U.S., touching the cheek of girls he thinks are beautiful with his finger, much as a housewife tests a heated iron. If the cheek sizzles she becomes a cover girl. ED.'"
-Ladies Home Journal, 1949.

manufacturers were making the latest fashions more accessible than ever, to every woman—wealthy or poor.

Where once mass-manufacturers had to steal designs from the top couture designers (like Christian Dior or Coco Chanel), now coutures began allowing mass-manufacturers to buy garments with the expressed knowledge that they were for copying—at a premium price, of course. Ready-to-wear creators unpicked these garments until they could be laid flat and used as a basic pattern; then they could be manufactured (often by simplifying a bit since the ready-to-wear industry could not hand-sew details the way coutures did). At a more expensive premium, buyers could get a *toile* or rough copy of the garment in muslin. Occasionally, special deals were even made where the mass-marketer was given an actual pattern—but only for limited runs. Even so, mass-manufacturers did hire their own designers (who largely went nameless and unrecognized) to create all-new designs in keeping with the popular lines and attitudes of the woman of the fifties and sixties.

By the end of the 1950s, many couture designers were suffering; mass-manufacturers were stealing away clients. Buying a mass-produced dress was far simpler (not to mention less expensive) than the old-fashioned couture method; the traditional couture route had for some eighty years been for a client to choose a design and fabric, then have their every measurement taken (the latter requiring at least 30 minutes of work). A week or more later, the client was asked to attend a fitting, then asked to wait again while adjustments were made. A second fitting was then required, and perhaps a third or fourth if the design was elaborate—say an evening or bridal gown. Though couture Hubert Givenchy once made a coat overnight for the Duchess of Windsor, the average couture garment takes two or three weeks to actually find its way to a client's wardrobe. Clearly, coutures realized, they'd have to modernize. While the old-fashioned methods were still kept in place (and, indeed, they still exist today), they were reserved for the most discriminating and affluent clients. For other customers, however, coutures soon began opening ready-to-wear boutiques. Still too expensive for the majority of women, and sacrificing most of the hand-worked details and all of the custom work that makes couture garments exceptional, these boutiques nonetheless gave couture designers an all-new market and succeeded in keeping them afloat while the ready-to-wear industry swept through the United States. "American women are always in a hurry," explained Mainbocher. "They want to pick a dress today and wear it yesterday." Christian Dior elaborated: "She prefers three new dresses to one beautiful one. She never hangs back from making a choice, knowing perfectly well that her fancy will be of short duration and the dress which she is in the process of buying will be jettisoned very soon."

Freedom In Fashion

"This is the new figure, the body line beneath the new mid-century fashions," *Vogue* explained in 1950. "You see an exaggerated bosom, a concave middle, a close hipline, a seemingly long leg..." Certainly the look of the fifties was all this and much more. After Christian Dior's "New Look" put fashion into an uproar in 1947, it wasn't until 1951 that an additional new style really took hold: the princess dress. Again originating in the Victorian era, the princess dress was cut in four or five pieces of cloth with no waistline seam; all seams ran vertically down the body. "The Princess has arrived! Long live the Princess!" *McCall's Pattern Fashions* magazine later exclaimed. Whether belted off to show a nipped-in waist, or gracefully clinging to the upper body alone, like most original "New Look" fashions, the princess cut made the upper body appear diminutive by making the lower part of the body wide.

Pencil-slim skirts continued to be fashionable throughout the fifties, but *The Picture Post* questioned early on: "Can anyone seriously contemplate hopping on a bus in a hobble skirt?" Designers listened, and soon the new slim skirts were made "moveable" by the addition of clever pleats and slits. "Because the leaves will be changing, so will the fashions," *Good Housekeeping* advised in September of 1950, trying to convince women they, too, could look like a fashion model: "This fall makes it clear, it is transition rather than turnover...The shape is a lean, lean shaft. Do not protest this too much, for designers have invoked all the laws of perspective to imply that you, too, are a willow want (and they've found ways to make walking easy, too!)."

Fuller skirts were often gathered into a waistband on less expensive dresses, while better designers realized pleating them into the waistband was far more flattering. For the ultimately flattering full skirt, the "circle" skirt was invented. Though its origin is cryptic, this clever style formed the skirt out of a single piece of fabric—literally a circle with the center cut out for the waist. Less expensive versions were created with two pieces of fabric and two seams.

Though bodices were essentially identical (form fitting), variations in necklines abounded. Sometimes simple rounded necklines ending just below the base of the neck, or scooping necklines (including necklines that plunged dangerously low) were worn, as were sweetheart styles and numerous off-the-shoulder variations. Perhaps most interesting were collars. Girlish Peter Pan collars were popular, as were Orient-inspired mandarin collars, and traditional pointed collars with flexible wire encased in them. The latter could be worn traditionally, or curved so that they stood partially up with the points heading directly down to the bustline, or, for the most chic look, could be made to stand straight up, pointing toward (and often beyond) the ears.

Pushing the bustline up as high as possible and dropping the waistline to the hips, Dior's 1954 "H-line" seemed well suited to a country that was preoccupied with the H-bomb. In 1955 Dior launched the equally successful "Y-" and "A-lines." With very large collars creating a top-heavy look, the Y-line was the complete opposite of most "New Look" inspired designs (which made light of the top half of a woman and emphasized her latter half). The "A-line," on the other hand, subtly reshaped the current bell-shape

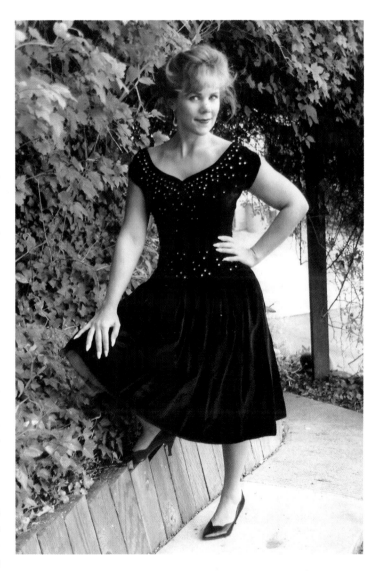

Reminiscent of stars shining on a clear, dark evening, this stunning gown of black velvet embellished with clear rhinestones emphasizes feminine curves. The skirt has an attached petticoat of buckram, finished off with a playful ruffle of scarlet crinoline netting. *Courtesy of The Very Little Theatre.*

into a more gentle, triangular "A" by flaring from the waist or bust. In '56 Dior launched tunic dresses—ahead of his time, they would be the ultimate fashion of the sixties. "A significant struggle is taking place in Paris," *Vogue* commented in 1955. "On the one side there are the designers whose achievement is to create clothes of so strong a shape that they look as if they could walk across the room alone...on the other side are the designers whose clothes are not superimposed on a body: they have no existence apart from it."

If Dior was the master of fashions "that could walk across the room alone," then Coco Chanel was the mistress of simplified clothes. With her "little black dress," this Lilliputian French couture had been the toast of fashion during the 1920s-30s, but had fallen out of favor and closed her salon in 1939. At the age of 71, in 1954, Chanel was disgusted by what she saw on the current fashion scene and re-opened her business. "A dress must function or *on n'y tient pas*. Elegance in clothes means being able to move freely," she insisted. "Look at today's dresses: strapless evening dresses cutting across a woman's front—nothing is uglier for a woman; boned horrors, that's what they are...these heavy dresses that won't pack into aeroplane luggage, ridiculous. All these boned and corseted bodices—out with them. What's the good of going back to the rigidity of the corset? No servants—no good having dresses that must be ironed by a maid each time you put them on." Again Chanel was fighting a battle against the corset and all that came with it—just as she had in the 1920s.

There was mixed reaction to her first new line, however. Little loose dresses and jackets were not exactly what women were used to by the mid-fifties. Nonetheless, *Vogue* praised her—cautiously. "The biggest news is personality news; Chanel's reopening," the editors wrote in 1954. "Her collection is the talk of Paris, with opinion violently divided. At its best it

An evening gown à la Grace Kelly. Of pink satin, the only embellishment on this dress (home made by Lily Ruth Teague and worn by a former Miss Oregon) is the beading along the neckline. *Courtesy of The Very Little Theatre.*

This playful cotton print day dress dates to the early fifties, and shows continued Mexican influence from the war years. *Courtesy of Flossy McGrew's.*

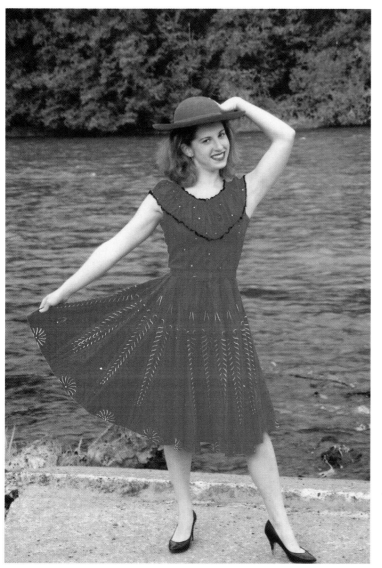

has the easy livable look which is her great contribution to fashion history; at its worst it repeats the lines she made famous in the 'thirties: repeats rather than translates into contemporary terms." This was very true, but, fortunately for Chanel, the young women of fashion who had originally worn her designs were no longer young and fashionable, and soon American women embraced Chanel—at least for part-time wear. "When in doubt, wear a Chanel," *Vogue* was soon advising—or a Chanel knock-off, we can presume. Chanel was also smart enough to follow the latest trend and open a ready-to-wear boutique; she explained to *Vogue*: "I am no longer interested in dressing a few hundred women, private clients; I shall dress thousands."

As early as 1954, the very modern, easy, T-shirt dress appeared. Quite literally a T-shirt made just long enough to pass for a dress, featuring ribbed cuffs and a collar, plus a belt emphasizing the waist, the T-shirt dress was ultra-modern, ultra-smart, and a look that lasted well into the 1960s. By 1955, the empire line was being revived. First worn in the late 18th and early 19th centuries, then revived with partial success during the 1890s, the baby doll look with the waistline raised to just below the bust had only minimal success at first—but would soon become the look of the early sixties. These first versions were usually in the form of long, slender sheath dresses which had been worn with many variations since 1950 (in keeping with the many Orient-inspired fabrics and dresses of the early fifties); sheaths themselves fit every curve of the body, not allowing for any bumps, but soon fuller skirts were worn with the empire waistline. Truly, the variety of fashion had many perplexed. Never before had there been so many styles and silhouettes to choose from. One day a woman could choose to look like a sleek rail, the next, she might prefer the look of a bell, while that same evening, she might choose a dress that gave her the simulated look of a little girl. "The tent or the hourglass, flowing skirts or tapering slacks—now we have clothes to suit ourselves, our types and tastes." *Vogue* tried to sort the matter out, and then concluded: "If we don't look our best, we have no one to blame but ourselves."

"Don't be a pin-up girl! Don't be a wash day pin-up girl! Forget the weather and the back-breaking toil of outdoor drying. Throw away your clothespins. The clothespin is the badge of a drudge! Modern women dry their clothes the carefree Hamilton way..."
- *Hamilton Automatic Clothes Dryers ad, Good Housekeeping, September 1950.*

Fashion magazines seemed acutely aware that women were confused fledglings in this new world of fashion. Guiding women to make suitable choices for themselves—rather than dictating to them in the old-fashioned manner—was the new quest of the fashion magazine. "It's a question of individuality in fashion," Vogue explained in their September 15, 1955, issue.

"And, the question is no longer how, at all odds, to achieve it. Now individuality is the fashion; the new clothes bring not just a single silhouette-change but several quite separate, smart 'new looks'...For some, its blessings are still disguised. For individuality—in fashion as in everything else—incurs personal responsibility. Though the new freedom in fashion is what women have longed for, it does mean this: more effort, more thought, and more knowledge, on the part of the woman herself...We sometimes hear, particularly before the big seasonal collections: 'I suppose They are brewing up some big new change in the fashion, and I'm going to have to throw out my entire wardrobe, thanks to your magazine!'...but, for the woman who's up to her times, the democratic new times make for wonderful dressing...as for saying, at any time, that this or that is the one and only dress-length, or suit-shape, or coat-collar, for each and every woman—never, as sure as this is Vogue magazine...Even the way a full evening skirt spreads itself—a completely individual undertaking, this season. In Paris, some skirts flow back to fullness from sheath-straight fronts; some big bells have trains, or diagonal tiers. And in the couture on this side of the Atlantic, full evening skirts make it practically impossible now for a woman to sweep into a room in a manner that isn't every inch her very own."

For the woman who wished to conceal everything, the sack or chemise dress appeared in 1957. The design was the creation of Cristobal Balenciaga, but—probably to his angst—Dior masterfully popularized the style. Though the chemise dress was named after the chemise dress of the 1920s, when created in true form, they were not at all alike. The tube-like dress of the twenties had been two panels of fabric stitched together at the sides, which hung from the shoulders without curving in the least toward the body. The new chemise, however, moved with the figure and gently followed the lines of the body. "Many manufacturers thought all they had to do was run up two seams, put a bow on the behind, and they had it," said American designer Norman Norell. "Actually, the chemise is a very difficult dress to make properly. The chemise is not a tube...It is supposed to be soft and clinging. Instead they made them for the summer out of stiff

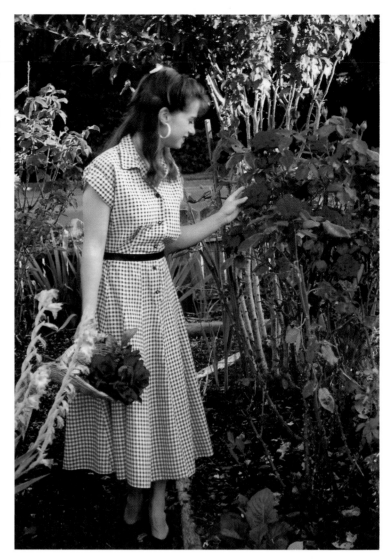

A typical cotton "house" or "at home" dress of the 1950s.

cottons. You saw those sights on the street that made everybody sick. Women didn't realize how they were supposed to look. They wore them too long. Also, they used an uplift bra, so that instead of falling against the body, the dress was pushed away." But whatever the original designer intended the new chemise dress to be, what was seen on the street was the popular fashion. 1957 also saw a brief vogue for "puff-ball" or "bubble" dresses. These were oddly arranged garments with fitted bodices and skirts gathered at the waistline. The hem of the skirt was then also gathered, creating a bubble where heaven-knows-what could be hidden from waist to knee. Another oddball style featured in fashion magazines of the era was evening dresses with slim-cut underskirts and fuller, flowing overskirts; these left the front open, exposing the slim skirt, but looked like a regular full skirt from the back. This style did not have great popularity when it appeared in 1950—but would be revived with slightly more success in the 1960s.

Steadily moving away from constricted, molded garments, Dior also launched his "Free Line." "The feminine silhouette changes from season to season," Dior said in defense of his constantly changing lines, "just like our habits and thoughts. Women dress for fun, not just to cover themselves." (No designer seemed to understand women better than Dior, and women publicly grieved all over the United States and abroad when he died in 1957.)

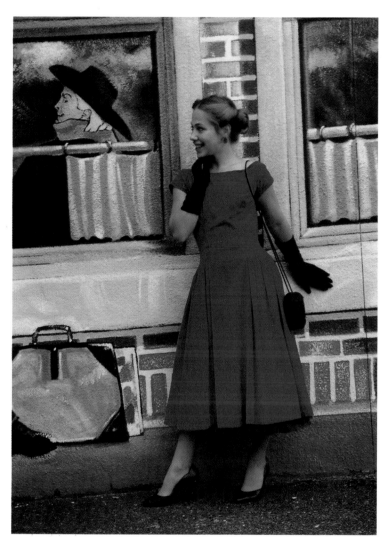

A flirty red velveteen party dress from the early 1950s. *Courtesy of The Very Little Theatre.*

Along with this new, less constricting style came a general modernization of dresses of every kind. Even the bell-shaped dress with a snug-fitting bodice began looking forward rather than backward, and a new shorter, less frilly look appeared. Looking much like a circus tent, the "trapezium" (or, as it was best known) the "trapeze" dress was introduced by Yves Saint Laurent in 1958. Many women adored it be-

cause—quite simply—it meant no more tightly fitted clothing—they could throw away their "waspies" and girdles, and not even have to suck in their tummies. Essentially, the design took the success of the sack dress and brought the loose style to its extreme. With a high bustline, and the back cut to fall free and away from the shoulders and entire back, the trapeze was an extremely large dress ending at the knees. Though some women relished in the comfort of this style, few even considered for a moment wearing it most of the time; it was, however, a popular style for maternity wear.

The "Oval" dress also appeared in 1958; it was essentially the sack dress, but with a balloon shaped back—Yikes! It was very difficult to cut and sew well (not to mention wear well), and was not readily adopted into mainstream fashion. Another take-off on the fashions of the 1920s appeared the same year: dresses in the simple chemise style, but with dropped waists and pleated skirts. The empire belt dress was also accepted widely by many women, as it hid a multitude of flaws. This style, also introduced in '58, was a variation on the trapeze, but with a belt just below the bust—the belt, however, slipped through the seams at the sides of the dress and clasped *under and inside* the dress, leaving the back to fall free.

Not everyone appreciated these loose, unstructured styles, however. In 1963, Bernard Roshcu wrote what he considered to be the general feeling amongst the male populous about this new trend. "In the spring of 1958 when women took off their winter coats, eager-eyed males were confronted by young women who looked like toothpaste tubes," he bitterly complained in an article for *Redbook*. "The view was infuriating. Fashion experts explained that the new mode was the 'loose look' or the 'relaxed silhouette,' but men would not be mollified. To them it was the 'sad sack,' the 'sag bag,' the 'waistless waste,' and a host of other epithets. So widespread was the uproar that Adlai Stevenson, addressing a meeting of 2,000 members of the Democratic party's women's organization, found time to comment: 'The source of the chemise is Moscow. Its purpose is to spread discontent.'"

In contrast to the increasingly loose day dress, by evening, dresses all through the fifties were the most constructed things seen since Victorian days. With fully boned bodices, padded if necessary to give ample roundness, interlined to ensure a smooth fit, and skirts interfaced with horsehair and Pellon, worn over full attached crinoline petticoats of netting, the look was romantic and Hollywood-ish. During the first half of the fifties, evening gowns mirrored day dresses: bodices were snugly fitted, and skirts ballooned like Cinderella's ball gown. Sleeveless and strapless styles

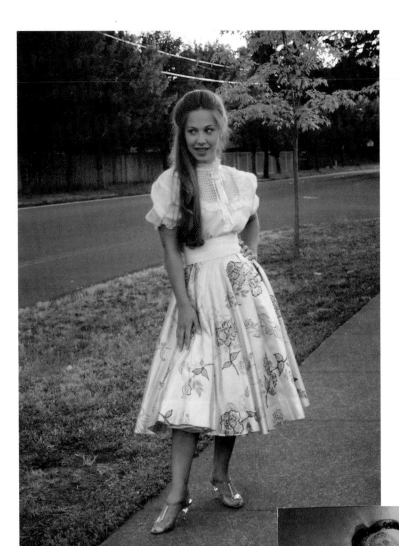

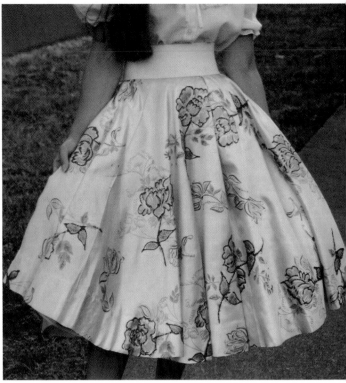

An Alex Coleman circle skirt of satin. The flowers are printed on the fabric and hand decorated with glitter. *Courtesy of The Very Little Theatre.*

prevailed. Skirts could be short, or long, according to the event they were designed for. By the end of the fifties, very fashionable gowns were cut short (just below the knee) but remained long in the back with a train, copied after Balenciaga's original model.

It was also in the fifties that teenagers were first widely referred to as "teenagers"—where they virtually created their own culture; for the first time young adults were no longer mimicking their parents—not dressing like miniatures of them. This is also the era when the teenage prom dress reigned supreme. Though still featuring the fitted bodices and full skirts of their mother's dresses, the fifties teenage prom dress was uniquely youthful—often made up in all-over lace worn over an attached, same-color slip of taffeta. Though net underskirts helped to make these prom dresses' skirts stand out full, separate crinolines were often worn additionally beneath them. To have a strapless prom dress was the hallmark of style (and of understanding, "hip" parents)—the look most girls pined for when their mothers insisted they wear a more modest spaghetti strap or sleeved style. Skirts—unlike many adult evening gowns—were usually relatively short, often ending at mid-calf or just under the knee.

"The full-length evening gown has returned!" McCall's Pattern Fashions proclaimed joyously. Though most women had worn full-length evening dresses in the first few years of the fifties (and indeed, in the 1930s-40s), the style had gone out of favor by mid-decade. Yet, McCall's noted, it now "returned with drama and magnificence not known for several decades." Whether the fitted and bell-shaped Cinderella gown, or the long and slender siren dress, McCall's wondered why "a fashion at once so feminine and alluring...[was] never missed from the evening scene?"

"Working Girls"

"Any time we girls have to go to work the result, historically, is that we do things better than the opposite sex," plucky Anita Loose, author of Gentlemen Prefer Blondes, wrote in a 1951 issue of Vogue. "I mean gentleman will go to all the trouble of keeping office hours and holding Board Meetings and getting Mr. Gallop to make a poll, and sending their Public Relations agents to Washington, in order to reach a decision which any blonde could reach while she was refurbishing her lipstick." Well, anyway, that was Loose's explanation as to why women were, for the first time in large numbers, staying in the workforce—even though the war was over. Indeed, it was such a phenomenon that whole new lines of clothing were created for this new market, and magazines were specifically created for office girls (like Glamour, which started out in 1939 as a pattern catalog titled Glamour of Hollywood, but, during the late forties, changed its course, dropped its patterns, and adopted the subtitle: "For the girl with a job").

Though the working girl might wear a slim skirt and simple, crisp blouse to work, the suit reigned supreme in the office place, just as it does today. This was nothing that was taken note of at the time. After all, women had been wearing suits—albeit inconsistently—since the 17th century. However, it does seem a bit surprising that women continued to wear suits considering that during the 1940s, suits were the practical garb adopted for lean war years. But, after all, suits were what men wore to work, and above all, women were trying to blend into the workforce (for fear if they didn't, they might be yanked away from their jobs as their grandmother's had after the first world war). Nonetheless, suits in the fifties were not unfeminine, and had changed considerably since the forties. Of the more important differences was the lack of heavy shoulder padding. Where forties suits had given women a football-player style shoulder-line, the suits of the fifties had much softer and feminine shoulders. During the first half of the decade, all suits featured fitted jackets, often ending just below the hip bone—a contrast to the war-era's usually boxy suits.

But there were other changes to be seen. When Chanel reopened and began peddling her ready-to-wear line, she brought with her a revival of her loose, falling-from-the-shoulders suit. "The heady idea that a woman should be more important than her clothes, which has been for almost 40 years Chanel's philosophy, has now permeated the fashion world," Vogue proclaimed in 1959. It was the same thing Harper's Bazaar had noted in May of 1954: "It is Chanel's premise that respect for the individual should dominate design; that clothes must be more important on the woman than on the designer's drawing board." It could be argued that Chanel's suits (and their knocked-off mass-produced sisters), with their boxy, angular lines straight from the 1920s, achieved the opposite effect. Nonetheless, after the fitted designs made popular by Dior, a loose, unstructured suit in Chanel-style must have seemed refreshingly comfortable.

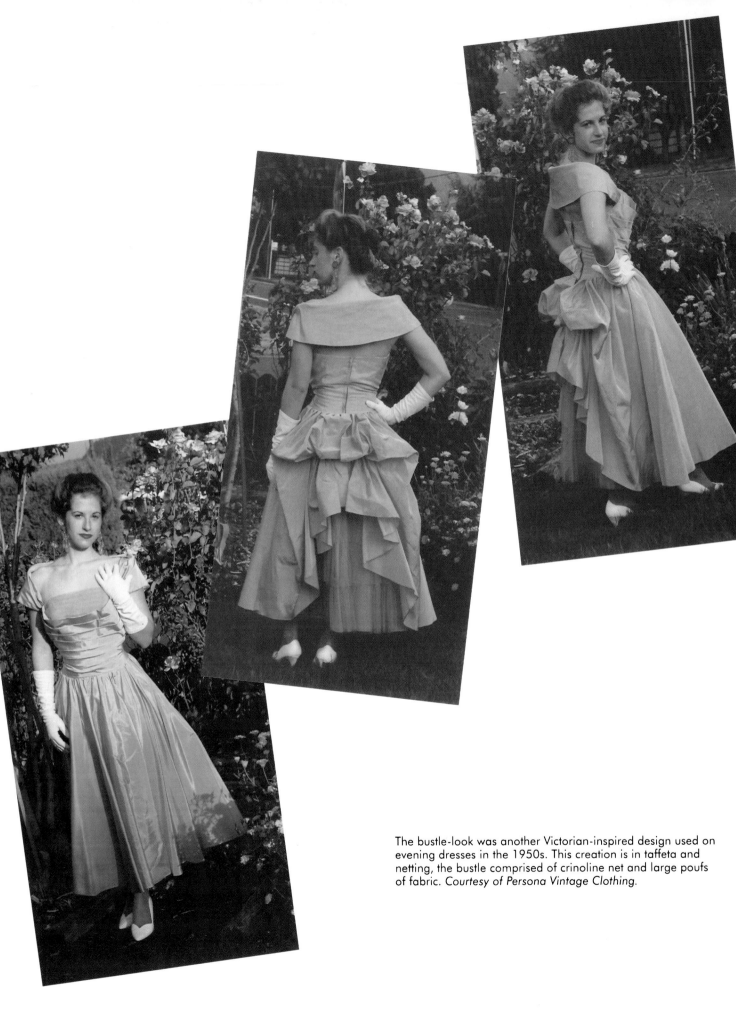

The bustle-look was another Victorian-inspired design used on evening dresses in the 1950s. This creation is in taffeta and netting, the bustle comprised of crinoline net and large poufs of fabric. *Courtesy of Persona Vintage Clothing.*

Dress & Undress

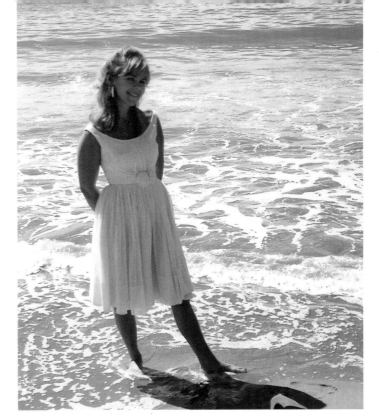

"What does fashion represent?" British *Vogue* pondered in 1959. "Decoration? Armour? A mood of society? For millions of working teenagers now, clothes like these are the biggest pastime in life: a symbol of independence, and the fraternity-mark of an age-group." It wasn't that teenagers had never worked before—indeed, they'd been a part of the workforce since the beginning of time. Rather, it was that for the first time, their parents were wealthy enough that the income the teenager generated no longer had to be donated toward the family income; it was, remarkably, the teenager's to spend as she liked. Manufacturers were quick to recognize this trend and capitalize on it. For the first time marketing directly to the teenager, the ready-to-wear industry created special lines for teenagers that were at once youthful, and—importantly—inexpensive.

Girls created their own look. As early as 1951, they were proudly donning saddle oxfords and poodle skirts. Originally, the latter appeared in wool felt or flannel in the circle skirt style, decorated by an appliquéd poodle on a leash. Later, the same term would loosely be applied to any circle skirt designed for teenagers. Beneath such skirts, crinolines were readily adopted. My mother remembers with great delight walking into department stores as a teenager and eyeing the racks upon racks of vari-colored crinolines lining the department store walls. Perhaps because, as my mother remembers, they were difficult to buy on a working teenager's salary, crinolines became a sort of status symbol, the idea being to try to hoard crinolines, sometimes wearing several under one skirt—the most fashionable girls wearing several colors at once.

It should not be thought that only teenagers donned crinolines, however. The stiff net petticoats were very much a part of Dior's "New Look," and had as much to do with the elegant Grace Kelly look as they did the frivolous teenage style. Ready-to-wear designer Anne Fogarty—whose early designs were marked by flirtatious dresses with snug bodices and full, crinolined skirts—noted that while crinolines were essential to the American look, in the early 1950s, they were still a rarity in Europe, and had a sort of gaiety still shocking to war-ravished areas. When Fogarty traveled to Europe in 1950, for example, she packed a dozen crinolines in a separate zippered bag. In Ireland, the customs officer took particular interest in this bag, and was skeptical when the designer explained that her petticoats were inside. In order to

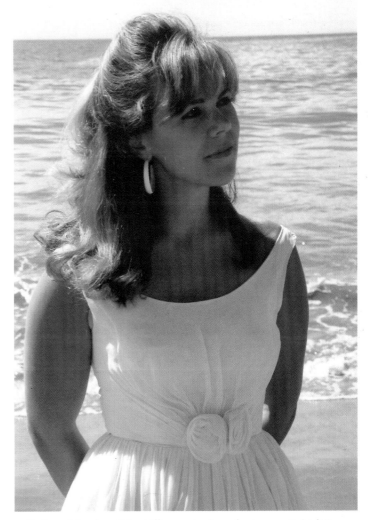

Soft and flowing, this chiffon party dress features a tight-fitting bodice and gracefully sweeping neckline. *Courtesy of The Very Little Theatre.*

21

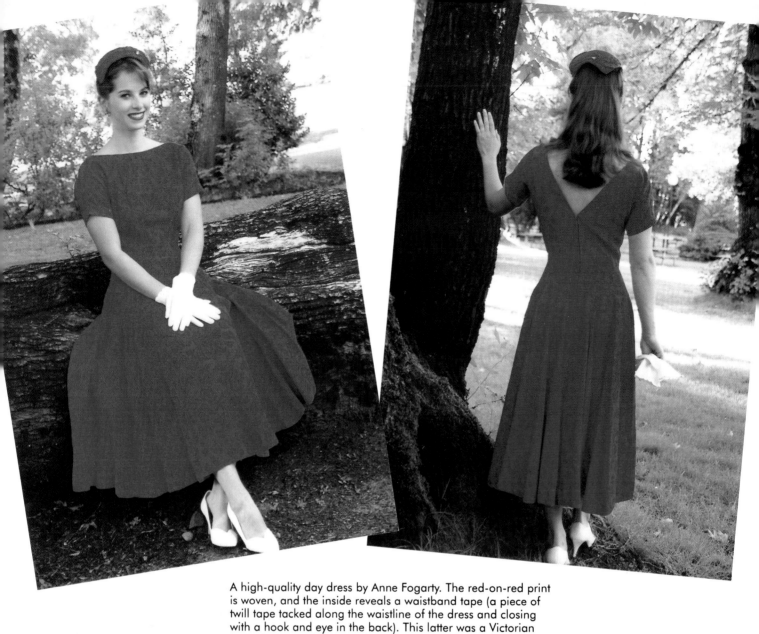

A high-quality day dress by Anne Fogarty. The red-on-red print is woven, and the inside reveals a waistband tape (a piece of twill tape tacked along the waistline of the dress and closing with a hook and eye in the back). This latter was a Victorian invention revived by Dior in 1947. While it made the dress fit better (keeping it from "riding up"), it was only used on more expensive fifties dresses. *Courtesy of The Very Little Theatre.*

reassure the man who peeked inside the bag and discovered stiff net poking out at him, Fogarty stepped behind the customs counter and lifted her dress just high enough for the officer to see the bottom half of the crinoline she was wearing. Though he may have felt himself a lucky fellow for such a viewing, he still insisted upon inspecting the bag and removing the petticoats—and soon full, colorful crinolines could be seen all around the customs office.

As tempting as colorful, frilly crinolines are for modern collectors, some care should be taken when shopping for them. To this day, square dancers covet crinolines for making their costumes more showy, and many modern crinolines can be found second-hand. It is often difficult to discern between an authentic 1950s crinoline and a crinoline that had a more mod-

ern genesis, but there are a few clues that will help. One is color; while certainly colorful crinolines were worn in the fifties, pastel shades and beige were most common. Size may also be an indicator; square-dancing crinolines are generally fuller than 1950s daytime crinolines (though fifties special-occasion crinolines could be extremely full). But perhaps the most telling clue is condition. Not only will modern crinolines be stiffer and glossier than ones from the fifties, but their elastic waistband will almost always be intact (whereas many 1950s crinolines have lost some elasticity in their waistband). One final clue may be the label. Modern labels are easy to spot once you're familiar with 1950s-style labels and their dated typefaces and logos.

Levi's, too, were considered hip—though they had been worn by some women for practical purposes since their inception in the 19th century. Still, the Levi's of the early fifties were, literally, blue jeans and only available in blue. Faded or patched Levi's were decidedly *unfashionable*—for, in the 1950s, if you wore them in anything less than "like-new" condition, it meant admitting you couldn't afford a *new* pair. Because traditional Levi's were still not made specifically for distaffs, it was fashionable for girls to wear a belt or sash around their waist to make them fit better, and roll up the hems of their jeans—usually to three-quarter length. My mother also recalls a particularly fashionable—if peculiar—style where one leg was rolled up, the other kept down. Though as late as 1966 *Women's Wear Daily* reported that in one women's fashion shop in New York City alone, 100 men's Levi's were sold a week to women (to be worn by women), if girls desired better fitting jeans, or jeans in other colors, denims were also available, designed specifically for women.

Teenagers were also the first to make modernized women's slacks popular. These included three-quarter length pants with zippers at the bottom to help them fit snugly at the ankle, peddle pushers (loose fitting, calf-length pants), and—a style soon readily adopted by grown women—Capris. The latter (named after the Italian island of Capri, which was a popular vacation area of the era) were more fitted than peddle pushers, and tapered gracefully to the ankle. That teenagers often choose to wear pants (especially as the decade progressed) was something to be noted. In 1959 *Vogue* did: "She's 18, and she chooses trousers because somehow one always seems to end up sitting on the floor in her room..."

Like Capri pants, women were soon adopting other teenager modes for their casual wear. Sweaters, for example, though never having been out of style, took on new significance in the fifties. Dresses were sold with matching sweaters; sweaters themselves were sold with matching sweaters: one pullover, and one cardigan, to be worn together. The latter could really be quite dressy, and were often beaded and made in cashmere and rabbit. "The sweater has grown in importance and size," advised *Vogue* in 1953. "Buy it two sizes larger than usual for a casual look. Add a sweater scarf, or fill in the V with rows and rows of pearls." A quintessentially fifties look.

Also to be worn with casual pants and skirts, halter tops appeared. Based on styles that first appeared in the 1930s, this scant summer top was mostly backless and featured strips of fabric from the front of the top which tied around the neck and held the garment in place. Likewise, a revival from the 1920s

also appeared in top designs: the middy. Roomy overblouses, often designed in sailor-style or in colorful prints featuring stand-up collars, they were largely favored for wearing over bathing suits, with shorts, or as cover-ups for scantier tops.

Too, a new invention rose to supremacy: the playsuit or romper. First worn in the late 1940s, and never to be seen again after the first few years of the 1960s, the playsuit featured dainty tops with shapely Capris, shorts, or bloomers, perfect for a lazy, playful summer afternoon. Sometimes skirts were added over them, but the design was always essentially simple, comfortable, and easy to romp in without worrying about revealing too much at the flip of a skirt (hence the bloomers).

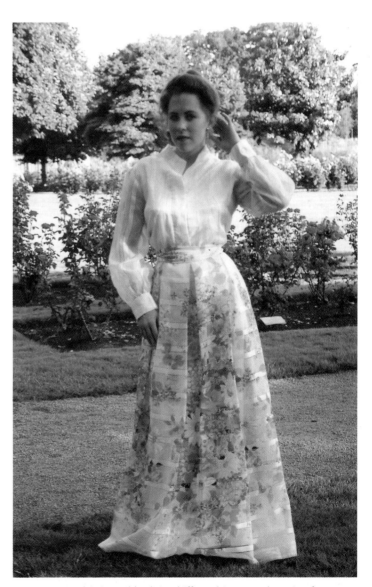

A more sophisticated look in chiffon, this party dress is of a classic style worn from the late 1940s up through the 1960s. *Courtesy of The Very Little Theatre.*

For modern collectors it may be difficult to distinguish between a playsuit and a bathing suit; even in the fifties the line between the two was sometimes blurred, and some bathing suits were made with the clear intention of not being swum in, but for lounging in beside the pool. However, only bathing suits usually featured built-in supports—often including light padding and boning. But whatever the case, swimwear itself was equally as flattering and graceful as the playsuit. "The bathing suit," *Vogue* declared in 1953, "has acquired a new state of—dress, not undress." While certainly women of the fifties were exposing more flesh than their grandmothers, most suits of the decade are modest by modern standards. Women weren't trying to flaunt flesh on the sand. The new suits never exposed too much—even when they were of the variety called the "bikini" (which only exposed about five inches of flesh between its top and bottom).

By 1955, however, a sexier look emerged. "Less suit's the idea—even maillots start lower on the bosom, stop high on the leg," *Vogue* revealed in 1959. Some of the most fashionable designs were strapless—but not meant for swimming in. (Sometimes straps could be added if the mermaid wished to take a dip.)

Improving On Mother Eve

The fashions of the fifties were nothing without proper foundations; all couture designers seemed to agree on this, whether it was Dior with his waist-cinchers, or Chanel with her *eau natural*, loose-fitting underthings, or Norell complaining about improper use of push-up bras. "Through the ages, women have

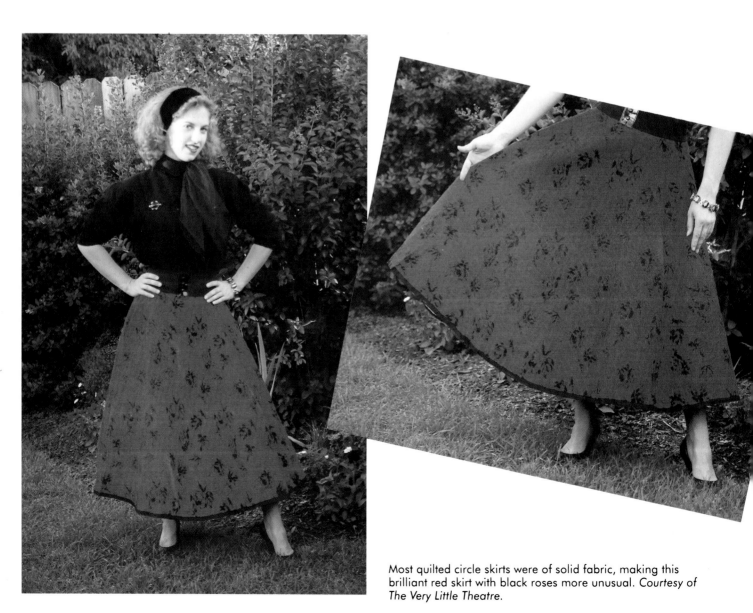

Most quilted circle skirts were of solid fabric, making this brilliant red skirt with black roses more unusual. *Courtesy of The Very Little Theatre.*

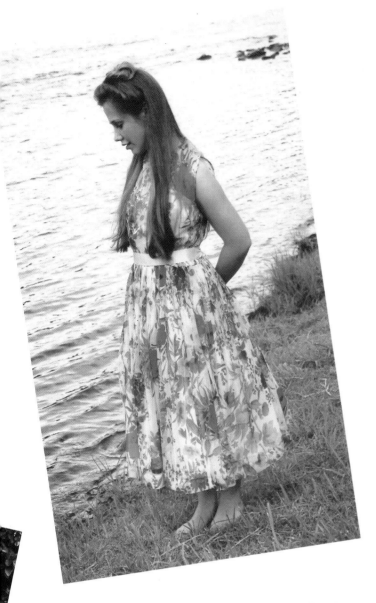

Colorfully printed with spring flowers, this 1950s chiffon dress typifies the soft, feminine look of the era. *Courtesy of The Very Little Theatre.*

always had a figure problem," a Lilees ad opined in a 1952 issue of *Harper's Bazaar*, "but there are new and wily ways to improve on Mother Eve *if* you trust to knowing hands.

"*Plot your fashion curves here and now, for this season's silhouettes are the most figure-conscious in many a year. They demand that your torso be fitted, but not exaggerated. Controlled, but free in movement. How do you accomplish this? Very simply...There's a revolutionary new girdle (patented) that takes inches off your hips, years off your figure. There is a girdle with no bones, no stays, no seams—a mere four ounces that makes all other girdles seem 'old hat.' There's a foundation too beautiful to be called a corset...such fabulous French elegance—with ribbons, lace, embroidery...*"

Every corset-maker seemed to promise such miracles.

Yet a good corset or girdle was exactly what every fashionable woman required, no matter how slender her figure might already be. No extra curve, no slight bump was allowed if you wished to be really chic. Incredibly, this revival of the corset was thought important enough that in 1952 a National Corset Week was created in England. Perhaps happy to see an industry that once meant booming business and dollars to the country, England cheered-on corsetiérs with fashion shows and excellent press coverage. By 1957, the importance of Corset Week reached its height when an inaugural luncheon was held so that expert corsetiérs could answer questions from the media about problem figures and their restoration with the aid of the corset. "There is," *Punch* (the English magazine best known for its satire) reported, "...fresh interest in the feminine silhouette evoked by Christian Dior...the most significant cipher since the S-curve of the Edwardian Gaiety Girl."

Still, most women were used to wearing some sort of corset or girdle—they'd been doing it for centuries, and the latest girdle seemed incredibly modern and emancipating compared to the old whalebone and steel cages once worn by women everywhere. "Fashions...seem to be made to order for the busy young wife," *Today's Woman* rationalized in 1953. "New bras and girdles have been especially designed for subtle control...the new American look from head to toe...Not so very long ago a corset was a monstrous thing made of whalebone, steel and lacing. To be in style a lady had to be nipped in here and pushed out there in ways that nature never intended. But see how times have changed...The new look features slim natural lines..." Well, maybe not so natural—but it was a step in that direction, and would eventually lead to total disregard for foundations by many in the 1960s.

Today's Woman was right about at least one thing, however; during the war, America had become the fashion leader. Now in the prosperous fifties, Europe continued to watch with a fascinated eye the uniquely American fashions that evolved in Yank country. Unlike the American trends that occurred (often out of mere necessity) during the 19th century, new American styles were now being adopted by Europeans—even the fashion-setting French. The French even manufactured bras based on American designs, including one dubbed: "*le véritable busty-look American.*" Though uplift, wired bras were often favored in the fifties, other bras might include foam padding, wadding, and spiral stitching. Merry Widow bras abounded; usually strapless, and always reaching all

"I never expected to see the day when the girls would get sunburned in the places they do now."
- *Attributed to comedian Will Rogers.*

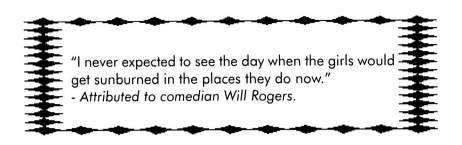

the way to the waistline, these bras were well-boned and gave a smooth line to the figure. Like many other fashions in the fifties, another Victorian style—rubber bust enlargers—were also advertised. All-in-ones were extremely popular, including bra, waist-nipper, and girdle in one garment. Sometimes even petticoats were attached for a maximum stream-lined effect.

Besides the corset or girdle, perhaps the most talked about underfashion in the 1950s were stockings. These had always been a favorite fashion article; even in the days when women's skirts completely hid their stockings, pairs were frequently made with very elaborate decoration. Nylon stockings were relatively new, however, only having been introduced at the 1939 New York World's Fair. Over 64 million pairs were sold there, but soon World War Two intruded and nylon was rationed for parachutes. Having been coddled and cared for carefully by women during the war, its little wonder that women were delighted to finally have stockings galore at their fingertips. Still, there was much talk about the durability of 1950s stockings. When they premiered, nylons had been advertised as "run-resistant," yet in the 1950s, women complained, they seemed to run at the slightest provocation. Were manufacturers doing this on purpose in order to get women to buy more stockings?

Good Housekeeping thought the issue important enough to run a cover story titled "The Truth About Nylon Stockings" in their September 1950 issue. "People say 'They're not so good since the war,' and 'Of course they're being manufactured cheaper to make us buy more,' and 'They used to wear like iron and now they fall apart in six wearings.' So *Good Housekeeping* decided to investigate." The problem, the magazine reported, was that before the war, old-fashioned silk stockings were treated with kid gloves because they were so delicate; women naturally treated their nylons the same way—first, out of habit, later because of war shortages. "Those pre-war nylons we keep rhapsodizing about were handled by us like crown jewels," *Good Housekeeping* reminded. In addition, they wrote, "pre-war nylons were almost entirely 30 or 40 denier. That means they were twice as thick and strong, and of course they lasted longer." But now, in the fifties, a more subtle, less wooden-

legged look was preferred, and most stockings were now woven in a more delicate—and attractive—15 or 20 denier.

Whatever the case, stockings still had to be held up by garters (almost always straps attached to the girdle), and were still seamed down the back. Seamless stockings appeared in 1952—but they were ill-shaped and bagged around the ankles. By mid-decade, manufacturers had improved upon this considerably, and most women switched to seamless stockings—except sometimes for evenings out, when seamed stockings suddenly became sexy.

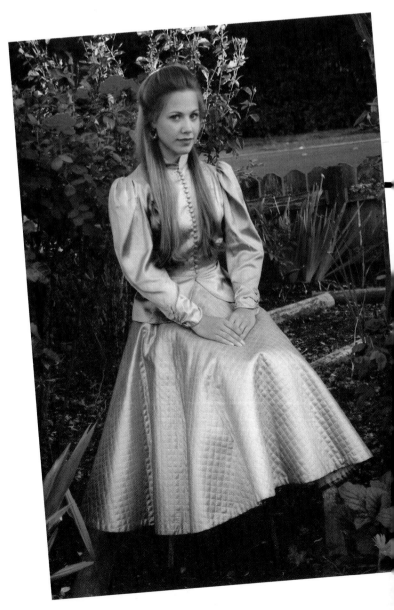

Million-Dollar Addenda

"But whether it's this suit or another, whether it's new or something you've had, remember that the final trick lies in the addenda...the little things that have so big an importance. The *additions*. Because it's really these that can make you look like a million dollars," *Glamour* advised in 1951. The look was well-bred, perfectly manicured, neat, and lady-like—and accessories were the key to pulling it all off. "You are essentially unfussed, pin-neat and organized," *Vogue* noted this return to lady-likeness in 1948. "This is the time of a muff or stole, a single touch of luxury to your city suit...immaculate small gloves...an exquisite tiny handkerchief unforgettably, fastidiously white."

Indeed, a fur stole seemed just the right touch for a fashionable fifties lady. But if she wasn't made of money, modern science came to her rescue. While the real thing was certainly preferred, it was perfectly acceptable to don something made of nylon or any other man-made fiber. Montgomery Ward, in fact, tried to hype the benefits of fake furs in their 1956-57 catalog. "Fashion's newest surprise, a truly miraculous achievement," they proclaimed. "Wonder fiber Orlon and Dynel, artfully blended and finished like a precious fur; plushy and warm—cleans like fur but needs no storage—it's moth proof!" If a fur seemed a bit much, a sleek coat, neat and fitted at the waist was essential. Or, if the lady preferred, a very full, cape-like coat might be worn. On warmer days, a little scarf tied round the neck was just the thing.

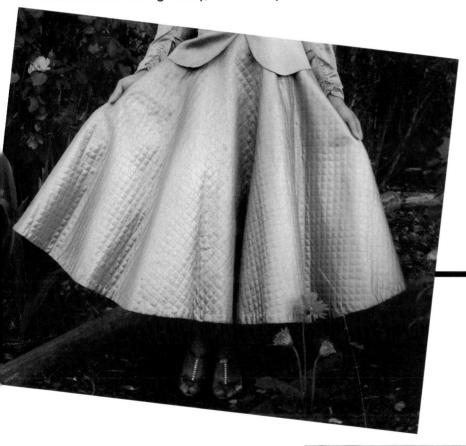

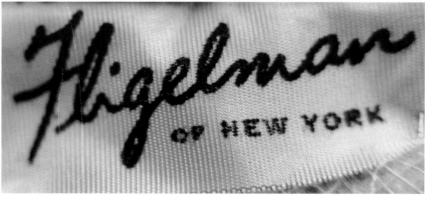

Quilted circle skirts were popular in the fifties among both young and old. The blouse is of satin with buttons and loops running all down the front. *Courtesy of The Very Little Theatre.*

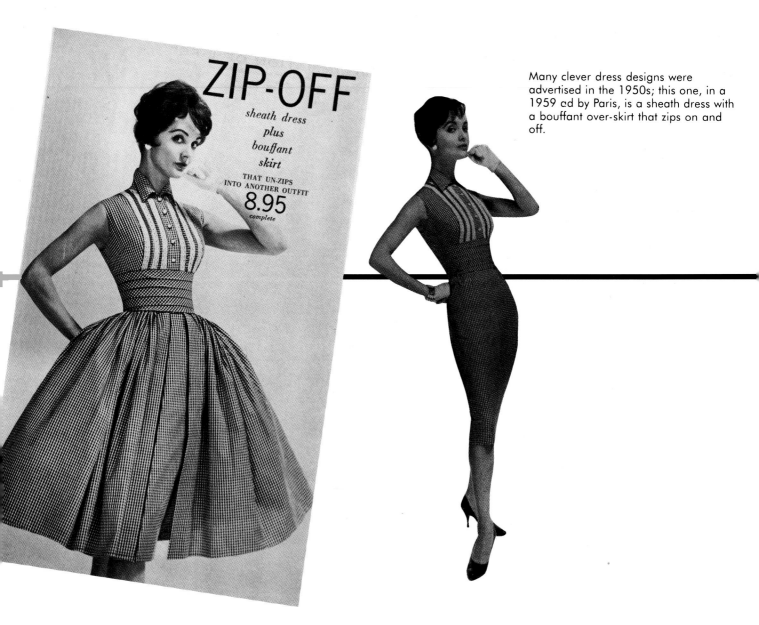

ZIP-OFF

sheath dress
plus
bouffant
skirt

THAT UN-ZIPS
INTO ANOTHER OUTFIT
8.95
complete

Many clever dress designs were advertised in the 1950s; this one, in a 1959 ad by Paris, is a sheath dress with a bouffant over-skirt that zips on and off.

Neither were shoes to be ignored. At the beginning of the decade, many shoes were still the clunky, thickly heeled sort worn in the forties. But by 1952, Dior introduced American women to the Italian stiletto. At first, toes were rounded, or even slightly squared, but as the decade progressed, relentlessly pointed and uncomfortable shoes were often worn. Other choices were available, however, including incomparably comfortable ballerina flats. Handbags, more than in any other decade, were supposed to match shoes perfectly if made of leather. Perhaps because this was largely impractical, many women sought out other sorts of handbags—including plastic bags. (The best of these were "Lucite," a trademark name for a type of plastic which gives interesting—often iridescent—effects. Lucite evening shoes were also popular.) Shaped in a variety of forms just like traditional handbags, these new, very fifties bags were nonetheless hard and immovable, with only the hard plastic handle having a bit of motion via the hinges that attached it to the body of the bag.

Gloves were not worn everyday as they had been in the Victorian era, but they were nonetheless essential to the well-dressed look. Black and white gloves remained staples, but as manufacturing methods and less expensive, man-made materials began to be used more frequently, many women chose gloves to match the color of their dress. Young women favored inexpensive, fun gloves in polka-dots, with beads, with flounces and buttons and bows. While most gloves didn't reach beyond the wrist, a number of dresses were created with three-quarter length sleeves specifically so longer gloves could be worn with them, and evening gowns almost begged for long gloves.

"Notwithstanding the continued practice of going bareheaded, best taste exacts that a hat be worn with street clothes in all cities whether day time or night," Emily Post insisted in the early 1950s. True, since the war, hats were not what they used to be, but most women still wore them for everything except the most casual wear. Still, most hats from the fifties are small and barely noticeable. Only hats that might be con-

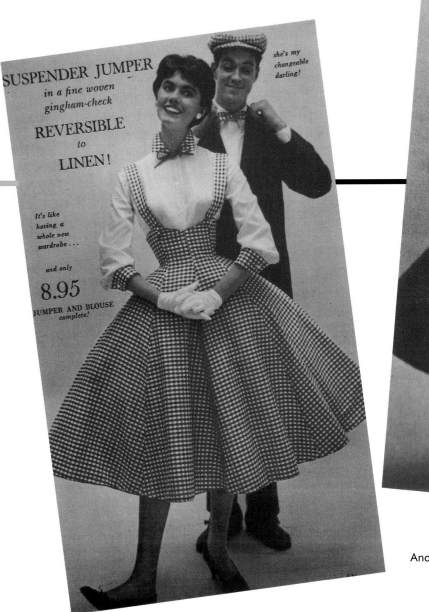

SUSPENDER JUMPER
in a fine woven gingham-check
REVERSIBLE
to
LINEN!

she's my changeable darling!

It's like having a whole new wardrobe . . .

and only

8.95

JUMPER AND BLOUSE complete!

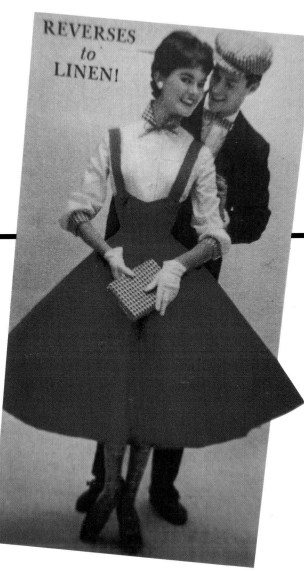

REVERSES
to
LINEN!

Another versatile outfit; this one, a reversible jumper.

sidered somewhat tacky are of any note at all. These were often trimmed entirely in colorful fake flowers, or—for a more classy look—genuine feathers.

The 1950s were the last years hats were essential to the designer look—and there were still a few hat shops and hat departments in stores like Macy's. Most hats were modified cloches, curved pillboxes, and "bandeau hats" (which were little more than headbands). Later, for the youth group, "ponytail hats" with a special opening at the center back of the head specifically designed for a teenager's ponytail, were featured in magazines. Wide brimmed hats were also popular—and considered important at the beach until the end of the decade when hatless was the only way to be.

What exactly lead to the demise of the hat is cryptic, considering that some form of the hat had been a mandatory part of fashion since the 16th century or so. Quite probably, many women got used to going bareheaded during the lean war years. Woman's new independence probably had little to do with it, since men still wore hats themselves. By the 1960s, the Pope began allowing women to go hatless during mass—for unknown reasons. Yet it may have been the milliner's own fault that her business was ruined. Lack of new and interesting styles and an abundance of ridiculous styles were probably the final axe to the millinery trade's head. Still, in the fifties, at least, etiquette books were still saying things like: "A lady never runs, [or] goes out of the house without a hat..."

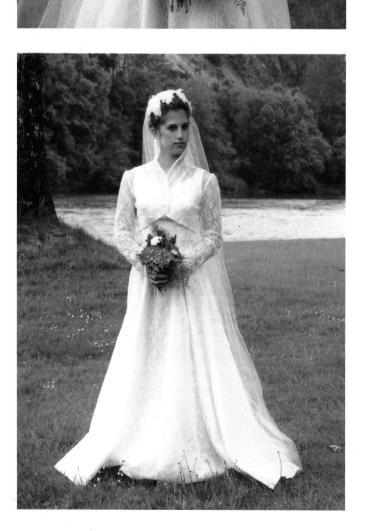

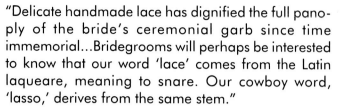
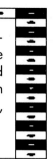

"Delicate handmade lace has dignified the full panoply of the bride's ceremonial garb since time immemorial…Bridegrooms will perhaps be interested to know that our word 'lace' comes from the Latin laqueare, meaning to snare. Our cowboy word, 'lasso,' derives from the same stem."
- Today's Woman, June 1950.

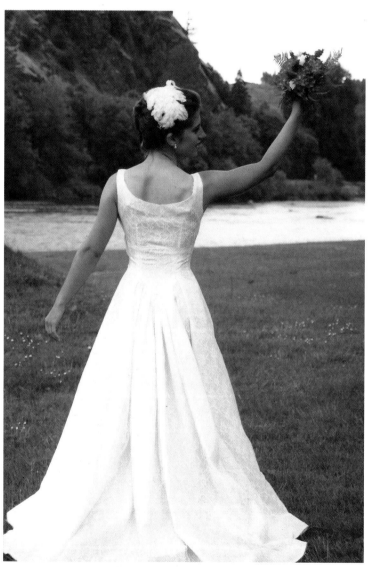

An all-over lace bridal gown from the 1950s. The dress itself is sleeveless, with a wide, rounded neckline, and was probably worn so at the wedding reception; a matching bolero with long sleeves and a standing collar with flexible wires provides the proper bridal modesty for the actual wedding ceremony.
Courtesy of The Very Little Theatre.

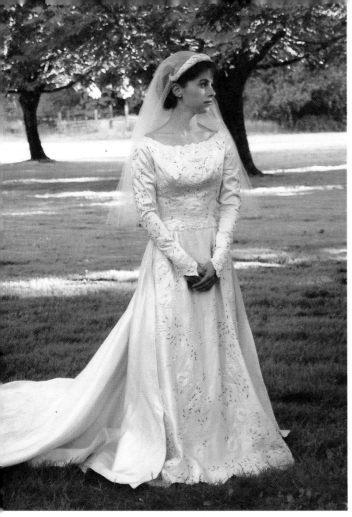

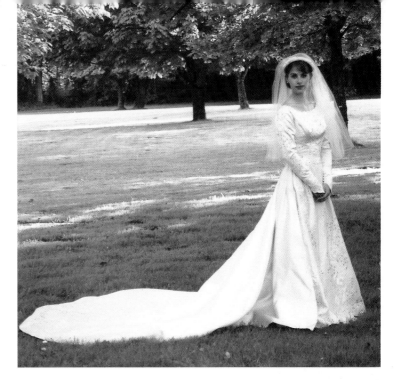

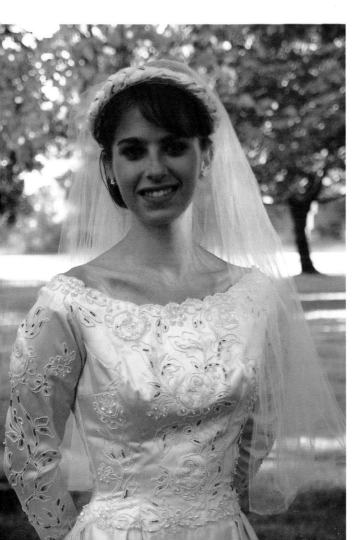

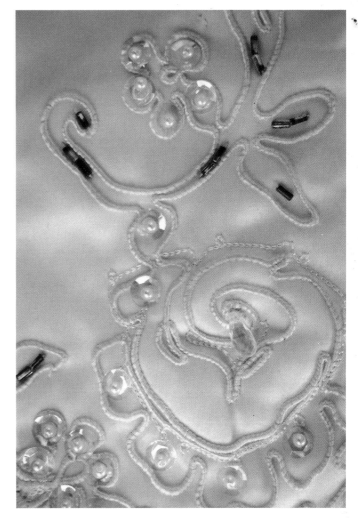

A magnificent bridal gown from the fifties, featuring a lavishly hand beaded bodice and skirt with trapunto (stuffed and quilted) details. The gown fastens up the back with some 30 tiny buttons and loops, and the train measures nearly 10 feet in length. The hem is stiffened with wide horsehair braid, and the entire skirt is stiffened with Pellon. The headdress and veil are of the same date. *Courtesy of The Very Little Theatre.*

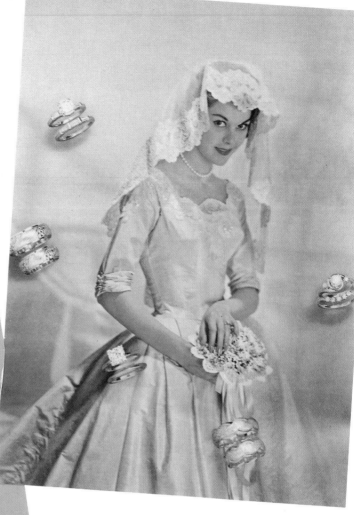

A 1959 advertisement for Artcarved wedding rings, featuring a classic bridal gown of the 1950s.

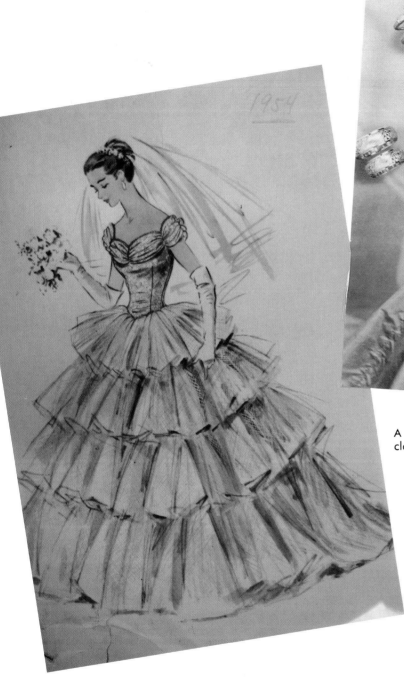

This Cinderella-like bridal gown is a copyright 1954 McCall's sewing pattern, requiring more than 50 yards of netting, plus lace, satin, and bodice boning.

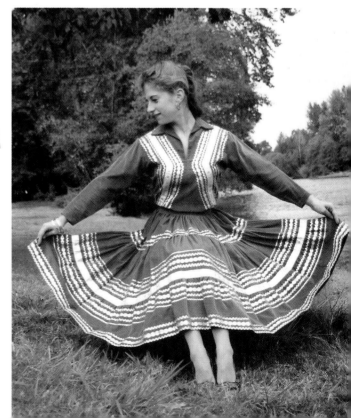

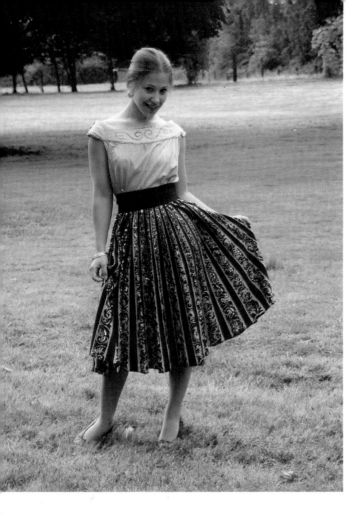

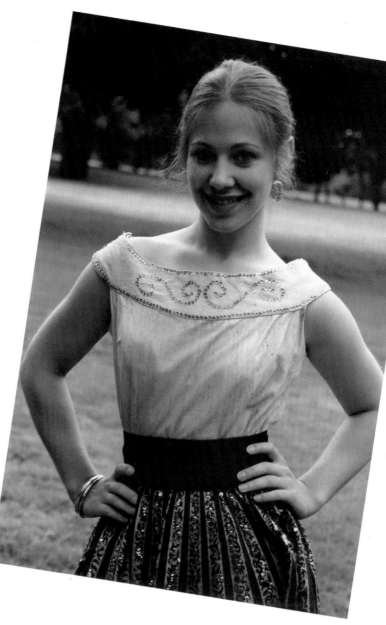

A "Made In Mexico" dress: the bodice is trimmed with pink sequins, and the skirt is decorated with gold sequins. *Courtesy of Flossy McGrew's.*

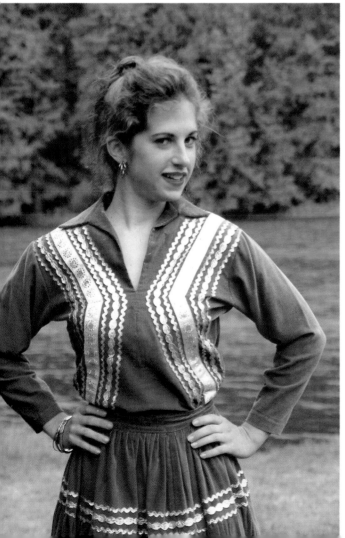

Mexican styles remained popular throughout the 1950s, especially in the early years of the decade. This two-piece corduroy ensemble is trimmed lavishly with silver rickrack and ribbon trim. *Courtesy of Flossy McGrew's.*

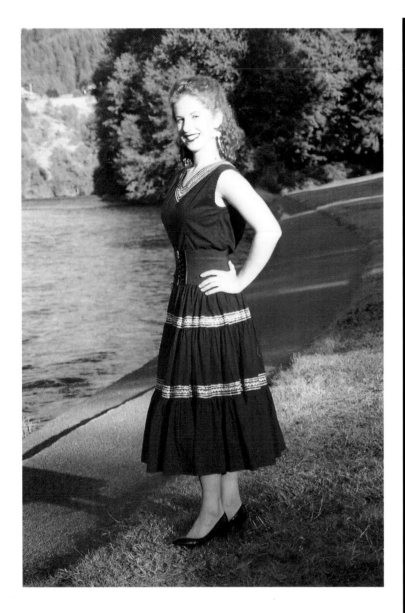

Another Mexican-inspired design, this one consisting of a bodice with a deep V in front emphasized by row upon row of silver rickrack. The skirt is in the "broomstick" style. *Courtesy of Flossy McGrew's.*

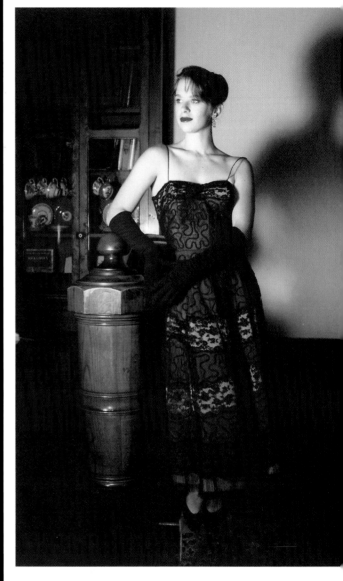

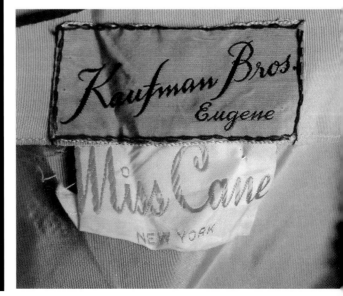

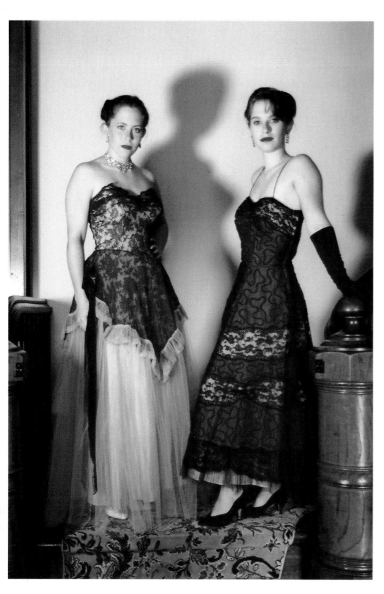

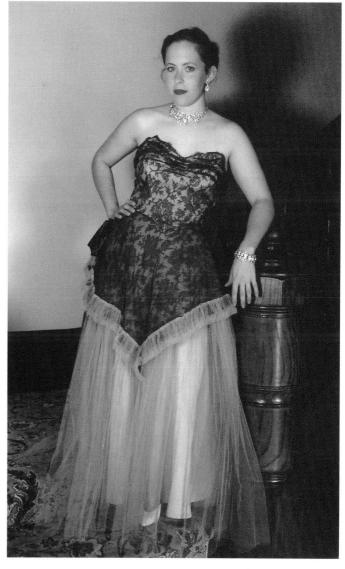

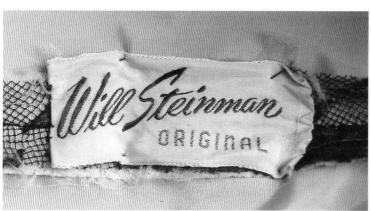

Two lace evening gowns looking as though they've stepped out of a bad Western flick. The blue gown is an elaborate concoction of layers of netting, ruching, satin, and black lace designed by Will Steinman. The pink and black gown has a pink taffeta lining covered with lace and netting embellished with black velvet soutache, and has a "Miss Cane" and a Kaufman Brothers label. Both gowns have heavily boned bodices. *Courtesy of The Very Little Theatre.*

A sweet summer day dress in a cotton print.

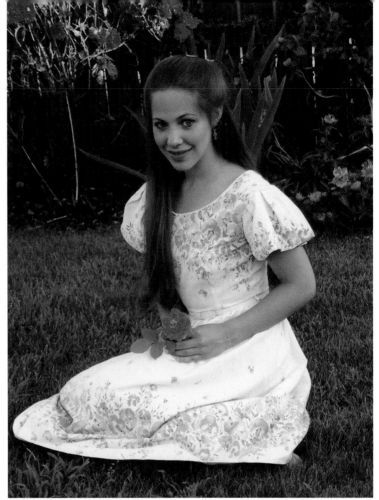

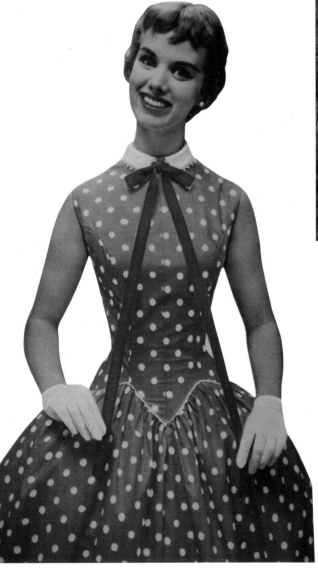

This Tenna Paige dress from a Best's ad was of stain-resistant cotton and sold for $10.95. The unusual waistline treatment dates to 1957.

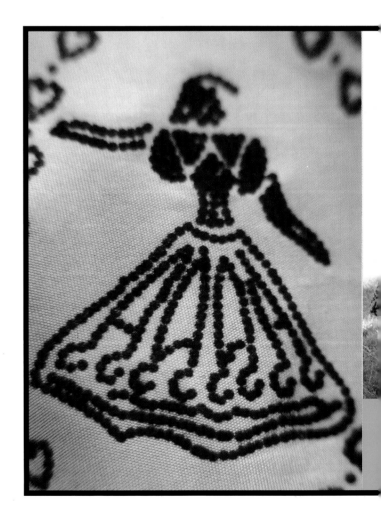

"Straw pumps and bags are the fashion, light in your luggage, right for silk shantung or cotton seersucker. The small cloche is the travel-perfect hat...Gloves are white corron or chamois doeskin, scarves gold and turquoise shantung, jewelry coral and turquoise beads, pearls and gold bracelets. Add brown calfskin pumps and a big barrel bag for en route, air-cooling sandals, white-linen or spectator pumps for destinations."
- *Ladies Home Journal*, 1949.

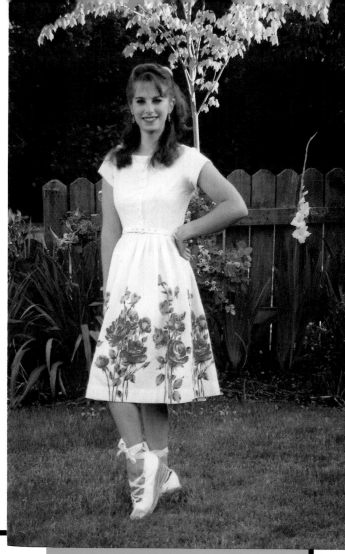

A heavy cotton day dress featuring a stunning rose-print border hem and a Montgomery Ward label.

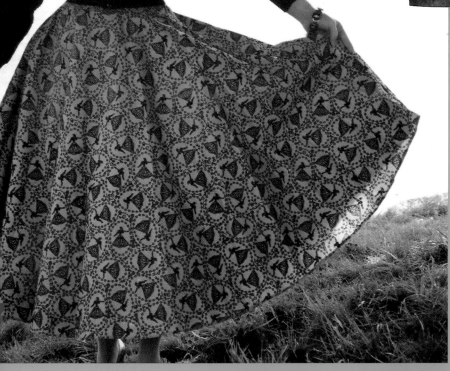

A paper-like taffeta circle skirt featuring ancient women in cut velvet, by Korday. *Courtesy of The Very Little Theatre.*

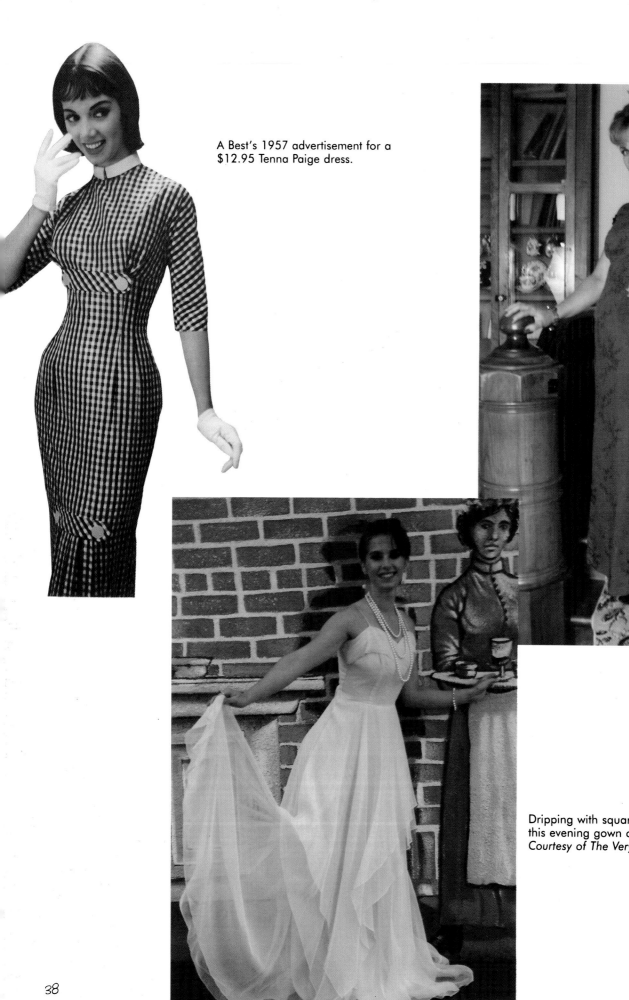

A Best's 1957 advertisement for a $12.95 Tenna Paige dress.

Dripping with squared layers of chiffon, this evening gown oozes with femininity. *Courtesy of The Very Little Theatre.*

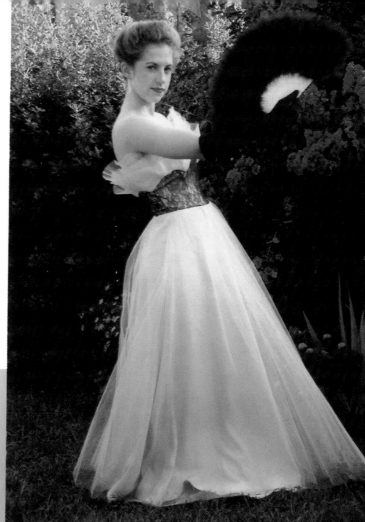

Of blushing net and black lace, this evening gown by Emma Dombe is a fifties fantasy. *Courtesy of Persona Vintage Clothing.*

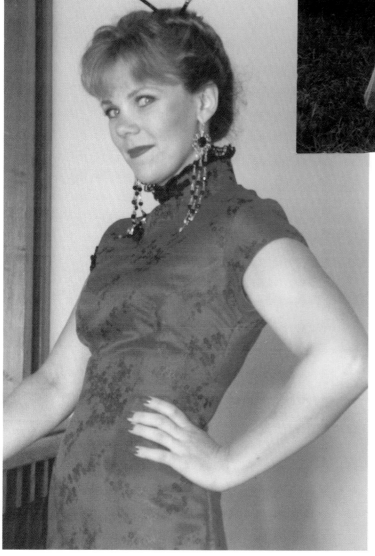

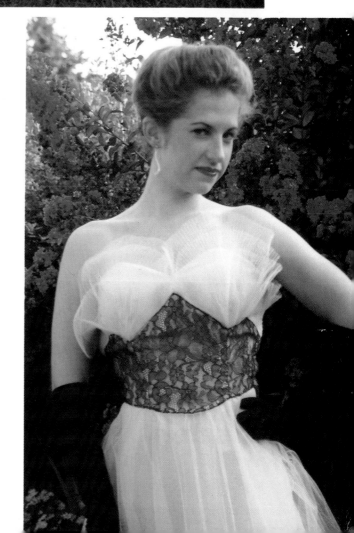

A slinky woven print satin Chinese-style evening gown from the 1950s. The slim skirt features slits up to the thigh, and the bodice is closed with black satin frogs. *Courtesy of The Very Little Theatre.*

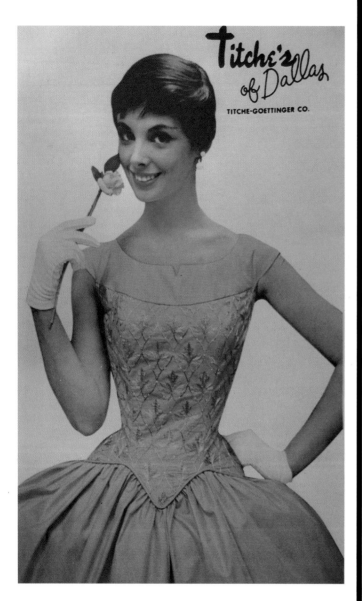

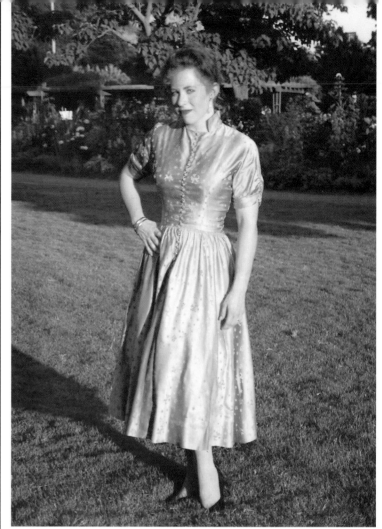

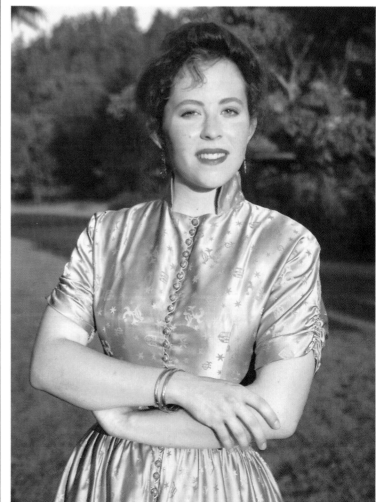

This 1957 ad sings praises for this Tenna Paige dress: "The torso look at its prettiest...with full, full skirt. Flower embroidery...Washable, crease-resistant lustrous Everglaze® cotton in mint, blue, pink, or lilac...$8.95."

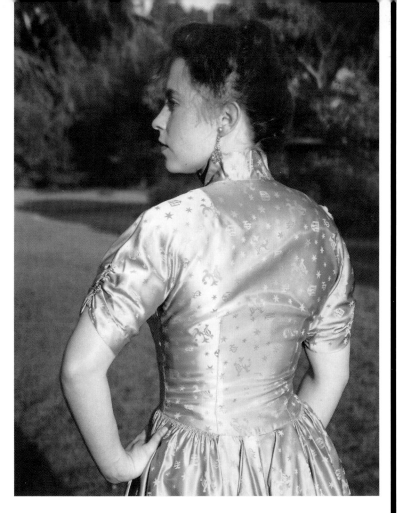

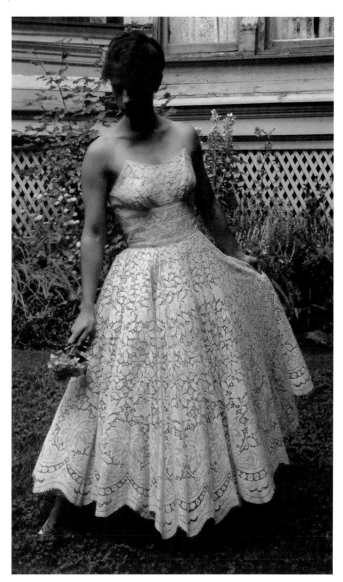

A fifties party dress reminiscent of the lace dresses worn in the early 1900s. With a full, wide skirt worn over a large crinoline, a heavily boned, strapless bodice, and a waistband lined in baby blue, this dress is the epitome of romance. *Courtesy of The Very Little Theatre.*

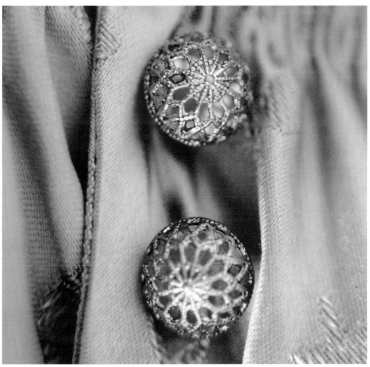

This Adele Simpson dress of weighted silk satin takes its inspiration from the Orient. Like most Simpson designs, the dress features exceptional detailing, including a gauged (hand gathered) skirt and sleeves, pinked seams, ribbon bound and hand-sewn hem, and hidden hooks and eyes in-between and under the glass and metal buttons. *Courtesy of The Very Little Theatre.*

41

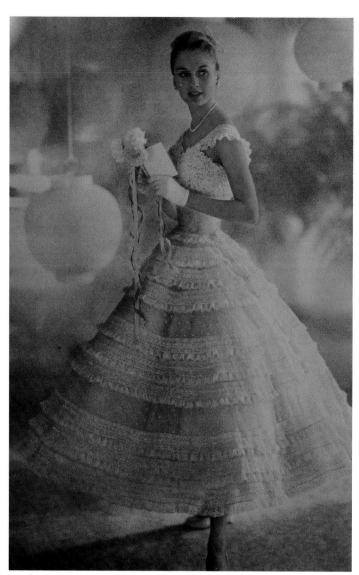

"'My lingerie stays so lovely with Lux care,' says Maureen O'Hara. Her favorite slip is pure silk satin in deep sulphur yellow with lace dyed to match...Its no wonder Hollywood stars insist on gentle Lux Flakes. These extra-safe suds keep slips and nighties enchantingly lovely 3 times as long."
- Lux ad, 1950.

Modess (a maker of sanitary napkins) had long been known for their ads featuring lovely ladies in gorgeous attire. By 1957, when this ad appeared, Modess and Vogue joined forces to create a sewing pattern for this dreamy party dress.

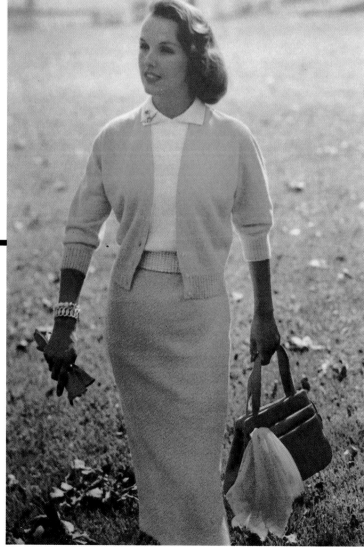

Never were knit outfits more popular than in the 1950s. This classic ensemble was featured in a Jantzen ad. Made of a lambswool, nylon blend, it sold for $14.98.

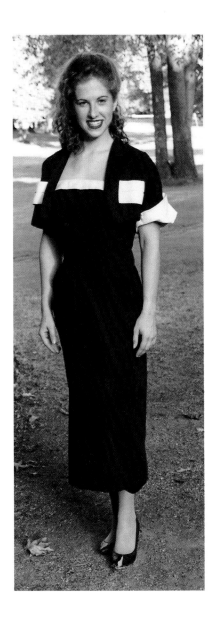

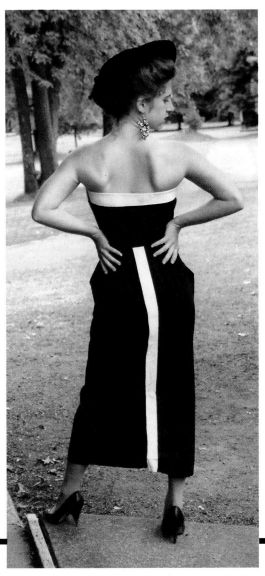

This versatile dress could be worn with or without a jacket, for day or cocktail wear. *Courtesy of Flossy McGrew's.*

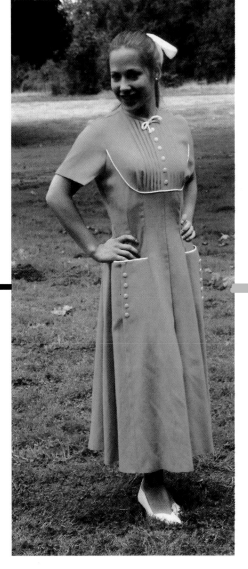

Not every dress in the fifties featured yards of fabric and lace. This house dress, like something out of *I Love Lucy*, is simple, but colorful and cheerful. *Courtesy of Flossy McGrew's.*

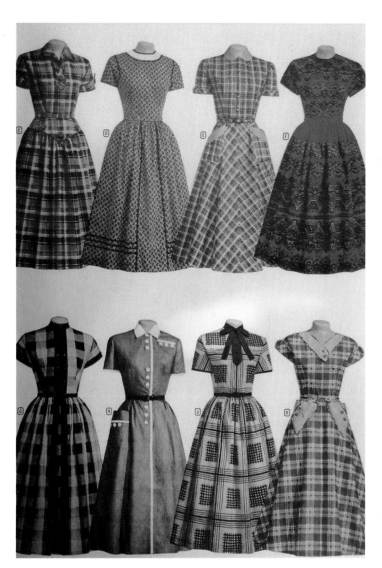

A page from a 1956 Montgomery Ward catalog, featuring typical day dresses.

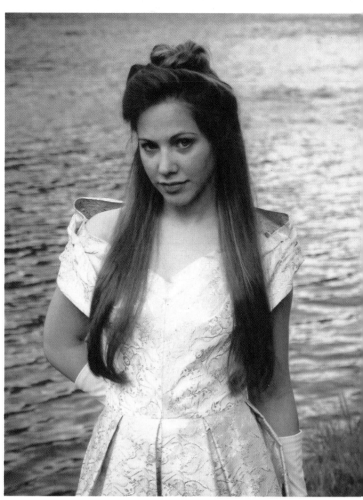

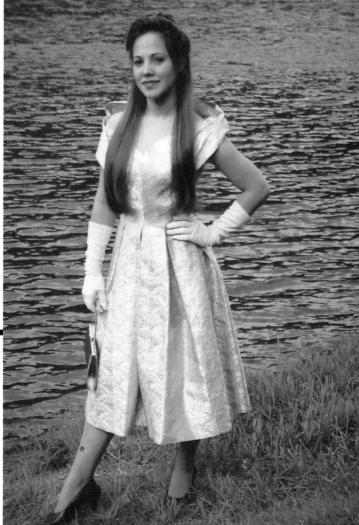

Of stiff metallic-shot fabric, this Modes Royale design features wide pleats and a large cowl-like neckline. *Courtesy of The Very Little Theatre.*

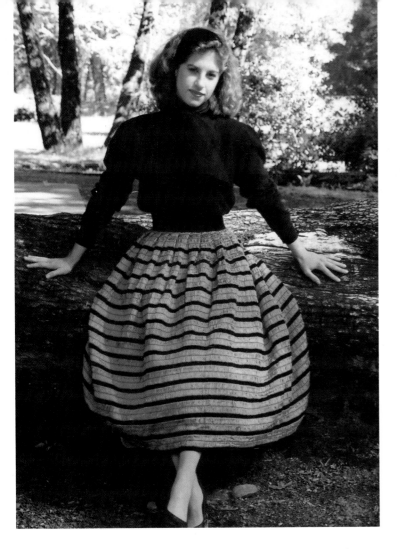

Made up of fine rows of paper-like taffeta ruching and black velvet ribbon, this skirt dates to the 1950s. The fashion for dresses and skirts made up of papery ribbons lasted to about 1960.

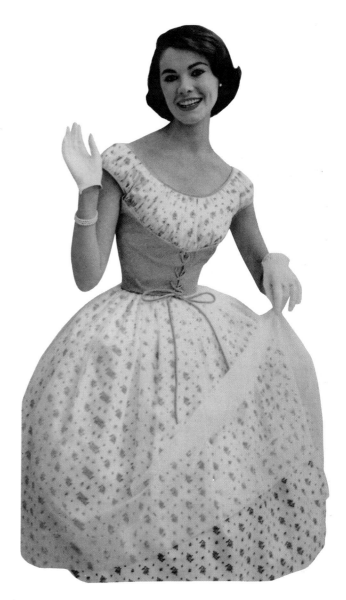

A 1959 Paris advertisement for a $10.95 "Shepherdess" dress with a lace-up corslette. This peasant look was featured in fashion magazines from about 1955 to 1960.

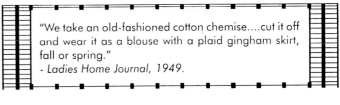

"We take an old-fashioned cotton chemise....cut it off and wear it as a blouse with a plaid gingham skirt, fall or spring."
- Ladies Home Journal, 1949.

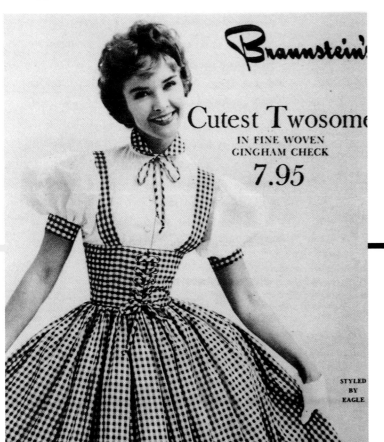

Braunstein's

Cutest Twosome

IN FINE WOVEN
GINGHAM CHECK

7.95

STYLED
BY
EAGLE

Another peasant-style dress, this one advertised by Braunstein's and costing $7.95.

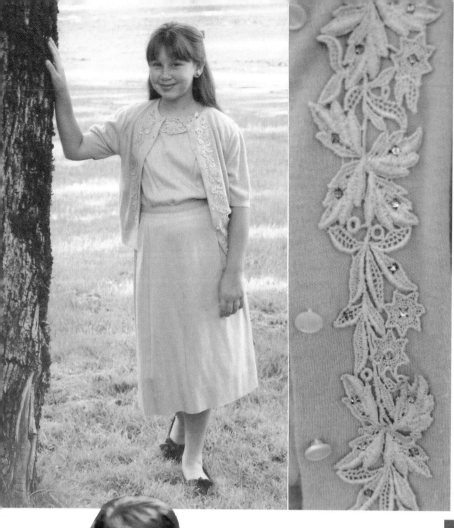

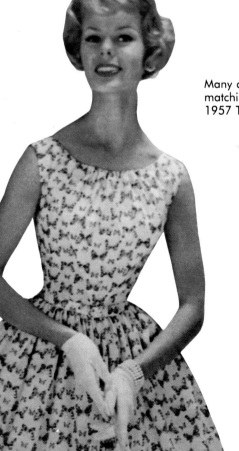

A day dress with a matching sweater, from the late 1950s. *Courtesy of The Very Little Theatre.*

A deceptively simple cotton day dress, showing expert use of stripes. The bodice is pleated and stitched down so that only the lace-like design shows, while the skirt is softly pleated, so that with movement, the wide stripes appear. *Courtesy of Flossy McGrew's.*

Many dresses could be purchased with matching sweaters, as seen here in this 1957 Teena Paige ad.

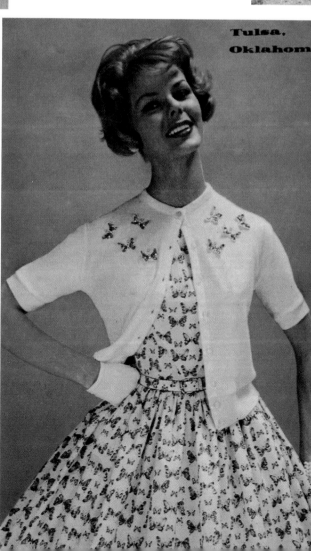

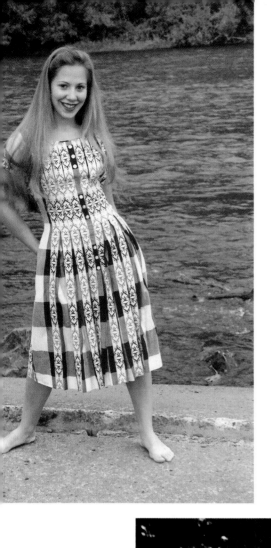

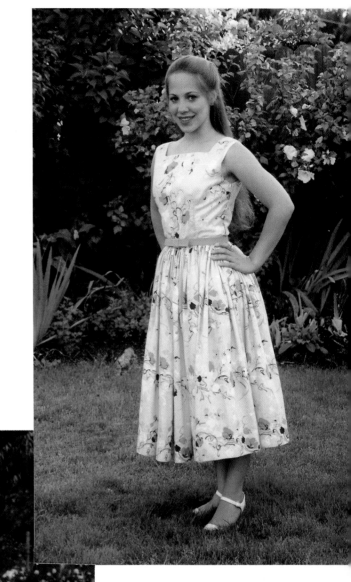

A simple cotton dress from the late 1950s or early 1960s. *Courtesy of The Very Little Theatre.*

A Spanish-inspired black lace evening dress with a snug bodice trimmed with poms-poms and velvet straps and bindings. The skirt is made up of nine rows of ruffles.

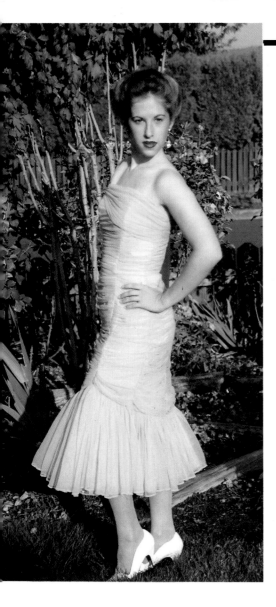

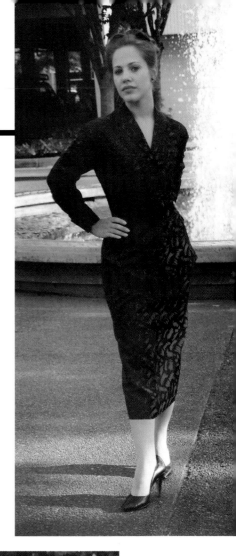

This sophisticated black and red suit is actually a dress (with a print skirt and plain black sleeveless top) and a jacket, meant more for cocktails than for the office. *Courtesy of The Very Little Theatre.*

This Emma Dombe evening dress could only be from the fifties! Of palest pink chiffon, ruched and pleated, and with a long, sweeping shoulder "scarf" of chiffon, this gown appears from the outside to flow easily—but the inside is boned to give careful shape and reveal curves. *Courtesy of Persona Vintage Clothing.*

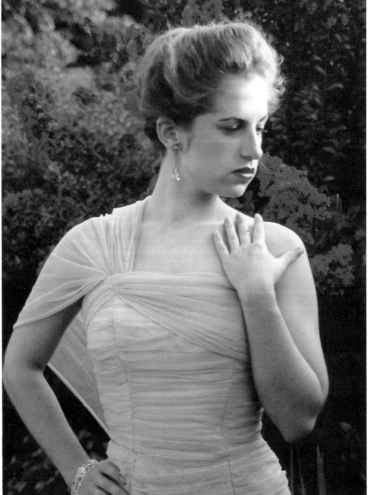

A darling suit, c. 1950, showing many hallmarks of "The New Look." The skirt is fuller than most 1950s suit skirts, and the bodice features a peplum and appliqué and beading along the collar. *Courtesy of Flossy McGrew's.*

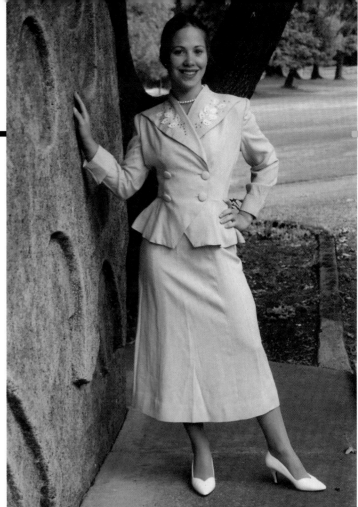

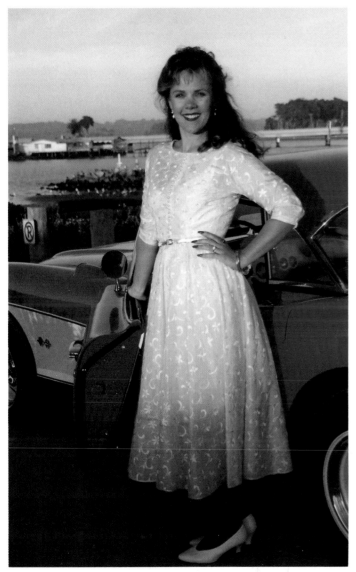

This cocktail dress shows clearly the basic style lines of most dresses of the fifties and early sixties: full skirt (this one is a circle skirt, and is therefore cut on the bias of the fabric and requires no pleating or gathering into the waistband), and a snug-fitting bodice. *Courtesy of The Very Little Theatre. 1957 Corvette courtesy of James Conn.*

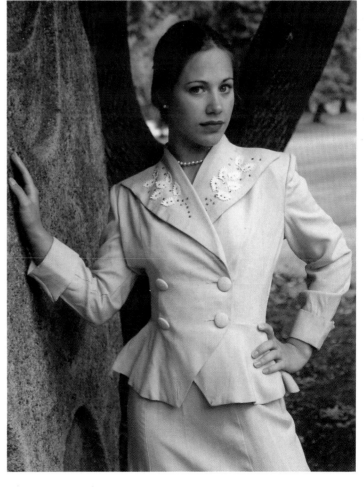

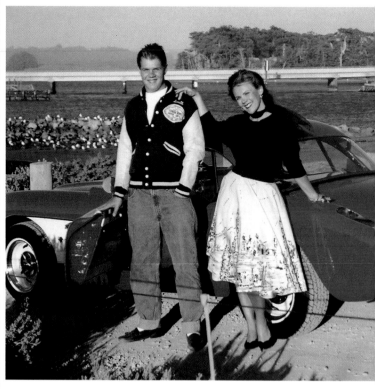

A hip duo: The young man dons loafers and jeans with rolled-up cuffs. The young woman also wears a typically youthful fifties style: A plain black knit top, a wide belt, a chiffon scarf 'round her neck, and a fabulous circle skirt. Skirts like these are growing increasingly difficult to find and are considered a collector's prize. The Mexican village scene is border-printed on the cotton fabric, but the sequins are all applied by hand. *1957 Corvette courtesy of James Conn.*

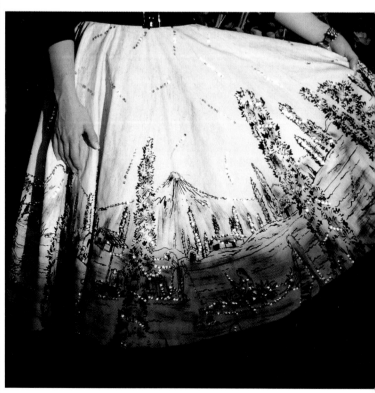

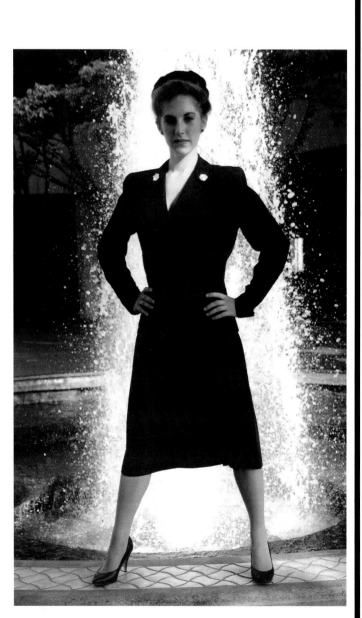

An early 1950s suit of black with rhinestones embellishing the collar. *Courtesy of The Very Little Theatre.*

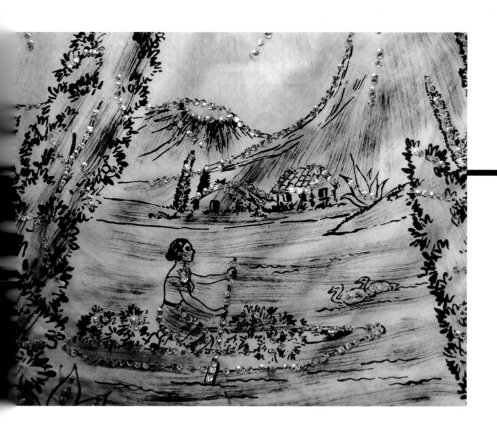

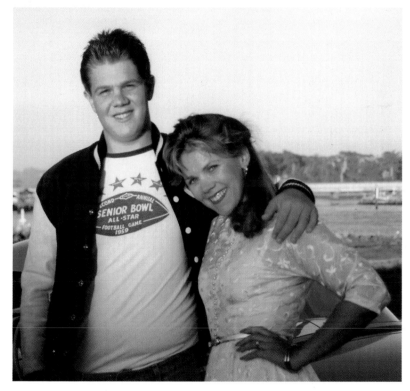

Varsity jackets embody all the youth and playfulness we tend to associate with the fifties, and, while still fairly plentiful, are popular among collectors. This jacket, along with the "Senior Bowl" T-shirt, date to 1959, when its original owner, Bill Dauphin, participated in a special (and short lived) event where four California counties selected teams to play at the Bakersfield College Stadium. *Courtesy of Bill Dauphin. 1957 Corvette courtesy of James Conn.*

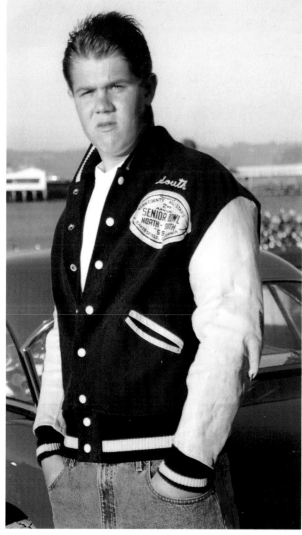

"Whether your figure is toothpickian, splendiferous or overly endowed, you can hurdle the girdle and look svelte without garter belt when you wear Suspants, the wonder undie. Wear it with garters to keep your stockings up or without garters on stockingless occasions...Rayon $1.50, Nylon $2.50. The undie you can wear with garters."
- *Blue Swan ad, 1950.*

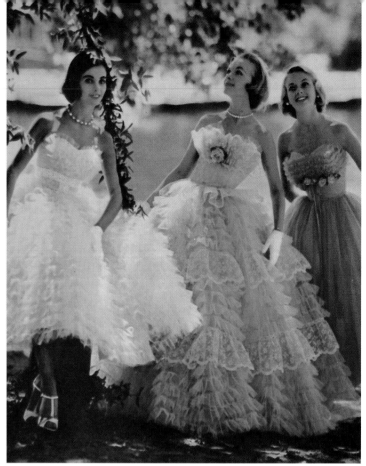

Excessively fussy, ruffled chiffon and net gowns were popular among teenagers for dances and proms. These were shown in a 1957 Nadine ad—a ready-to-wear company specializing in teenage formals.

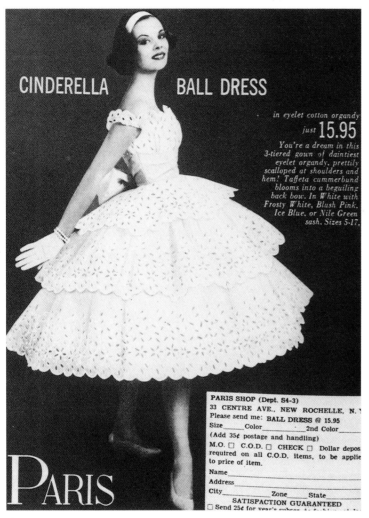

CINDERELLA BALL DRESS

in eyelet cotton organdy
just **15.95**

You're a dream in this 3-tiered gown of daintiest eyelet organdy, prettily scalloped at shoulders and hem! Taffeta cummerbund blooms into a beguiling back bow. In White with Frosty White, Blush Pink, Ice Blue, or Nile Green sash. Sizes 5-17.

PARIS SHOP (Dept. S4-3)
33 CENTRE AVE., NEW ROCHELLE, N. Y.
Please send me: BALL DRESS @ 15.95
Size_____ Color_____ 2nd Color_____
(Add 35¢ postage and handling)
M.O. ☐ C.O.D. ☐ CHECK ☐ Dollar depos
required on all C.O.D. items, to be applie
to price of item.
Name_____
Address_____
City_____ Zone____ State_____
SATISFACTION GUARANTEED
☐ Send 25¢ for year's subscr. to fashion-al b

PARIS

From a 1960 issue of *Seventeen*, a Paris ad for a lavish, eyelet organdy dress with a blush pink taffeta sash—$15.95.

A prom dress of pink taffeta and netting, with its bosom covered with silk roses. In 1951's *A Place In The Sun*, Elizabeth Taylor wore a white dress much like this—but with the bosom encrusted with tiny white flowers. The popularity of this film inspired hundreds of young women to don ready-made versions to the prom, and this pink dress is only a slightly-changed version of Ms. Taylor's popular style. *Courtesy of The Very Little Theatre.*

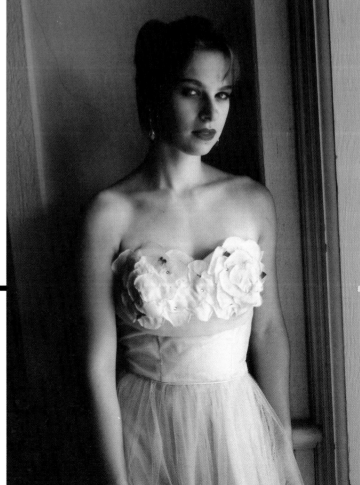

A teenage party ensemble. The bodice is of acetate, trimmed with ruffles, lace, and ribbons. The skirt is of papery taffeta, with insertions of chiffon, and the entire skirt is speckled with shades of pink "confetti," or "paint splatters." *Courtesy of The Very Little Theatre.*

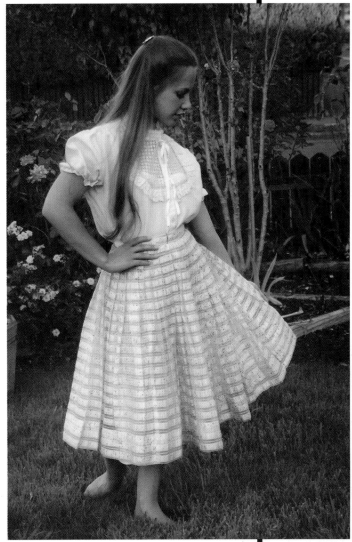

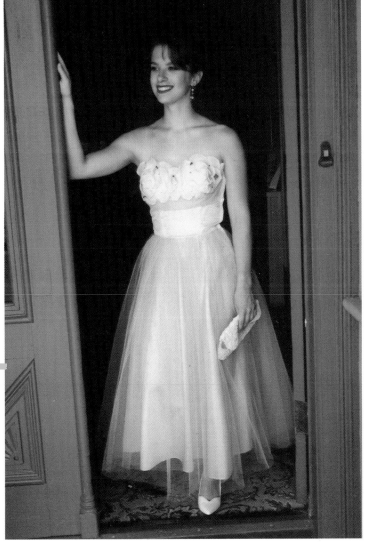

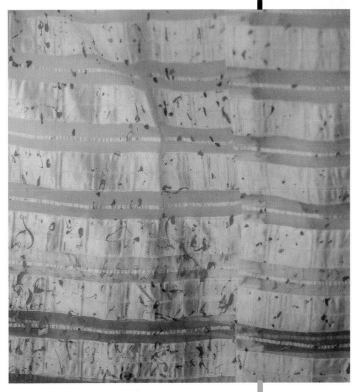

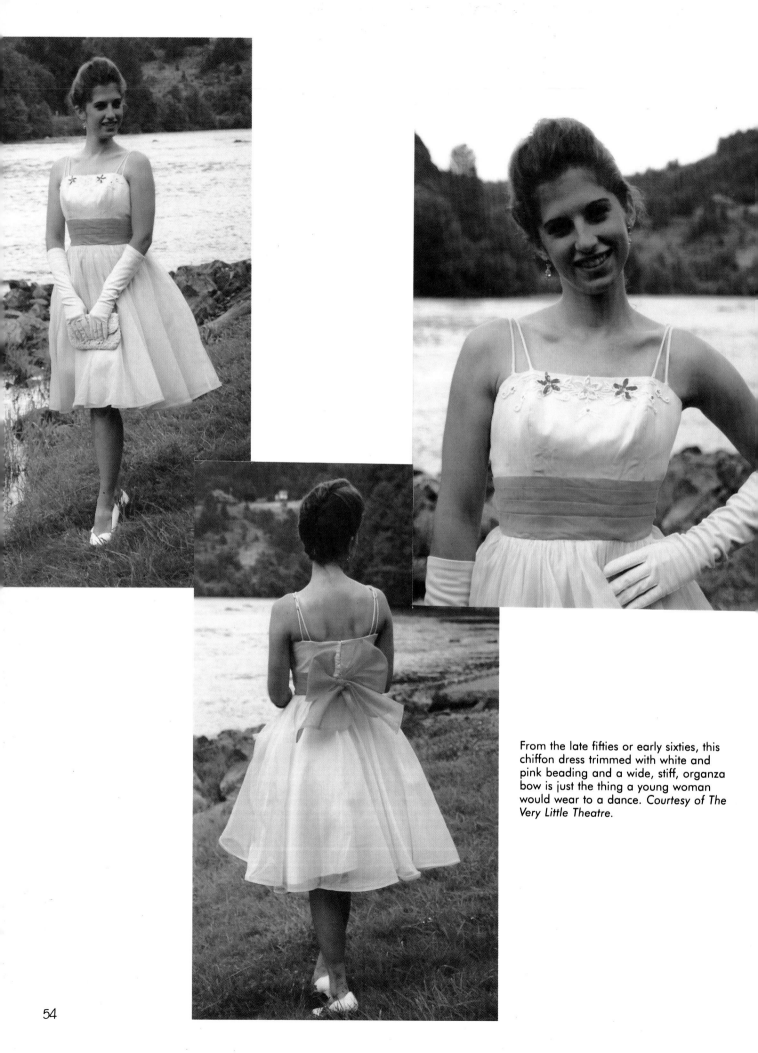

From the late fifties or early sixties, this chiffon dress trimmed with white and pink beading and a wide, stiff, organza bow is just the thing a young woman would wear to a dance. *Courtesy of The Very Little Theatre.*

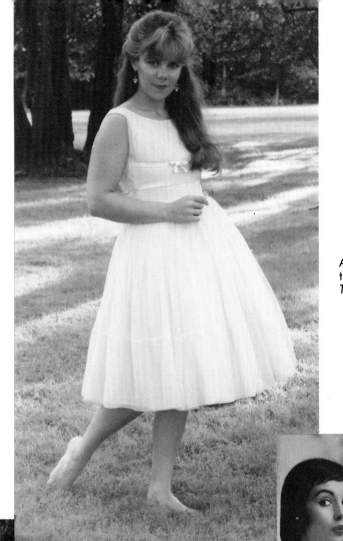

A dainty yellow chiffon prom dress from the fifties. *Courtesy of The Very Little Theatre.*

A Lord & Taylor ad for a $22.95 Jonathan Logan ensemble.

Jonathan Logan

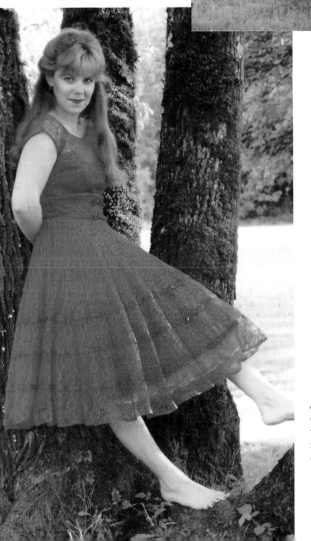

A 1950s prom dress of all-over red lace, featuring bands of satin ribbon and bows along the hemline and bodice.

A Paris ad for a nautically inspired teenage dress of red corduroy.

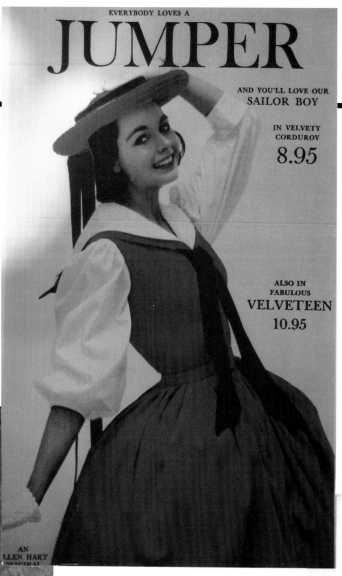

EVERYBODY LOVES A
JUMPER
AND YOU'LL LOVE OUR
SAILOR BOY

IN VELVETY
CORDUROY
8.95

ALSO IN
FABULOUS
VELVETEEN
10.95

AN
LLEN HART
RIGINAL

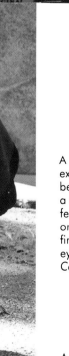

A "poodle skirt" of felt. It can be exceedingly difficult to distinguish between an authentic poodle skirt and a costume or reproduction, but this skirt features all the hallmarks of an original: a metal zipper, carefully finished edges, fine details, a hook and eye waistband, and hanger loops. *Courtesy of The Very Little Theatre.*

A young teenager's school dress in traditional plaid with a black velvet collar and wide black belt. *Courtesy of The Very Little Theatre.*

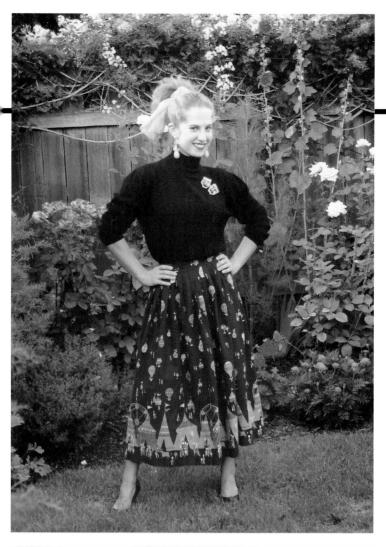

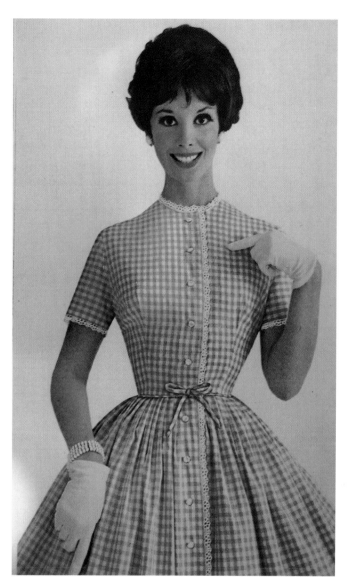

A Tenna Paige advertisement from 1960, featuring a simple gingham dress for $11.98.

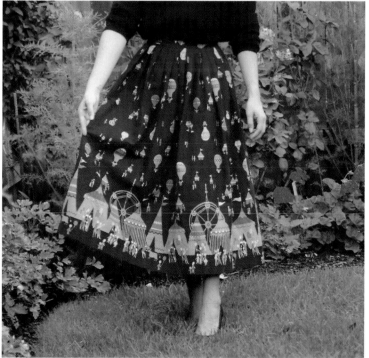

Cotton skirts with border prints were very popular in the fifties, but are difficult to find today. This cotton version depicts of a fair, with a multitude of fair goers flying in hot air balloons. The color scheme dates it to the late 1950s or early 1960s.

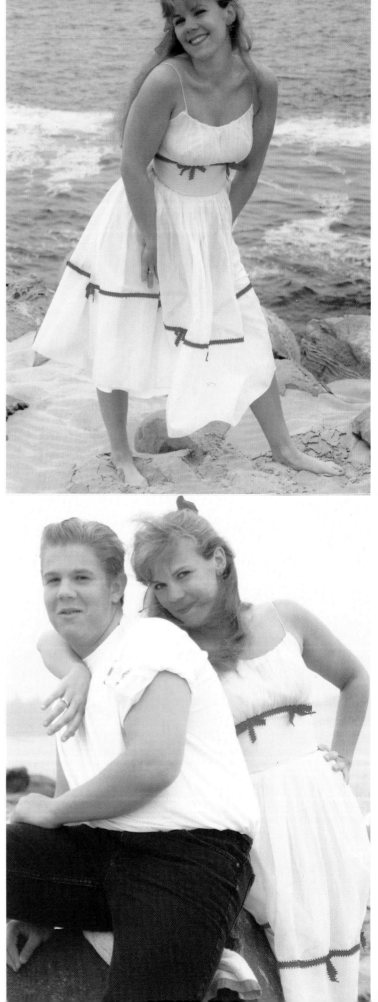

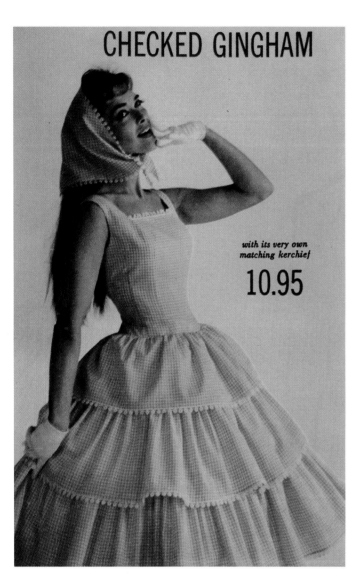

CHECKED GINGHAM

with its very own matching kerchief

10.95

Though traditional ginghams were in fashion all through the 1950s and early 1960s, baby blue and pink gingham dresses were heavily featured in fashion magazines the summer of 1960. This Paris ad featured an ultra-feminine gingham for $10.95.

A girlish chiffon party dress punctuated with dainty red picot ribbon and bows.

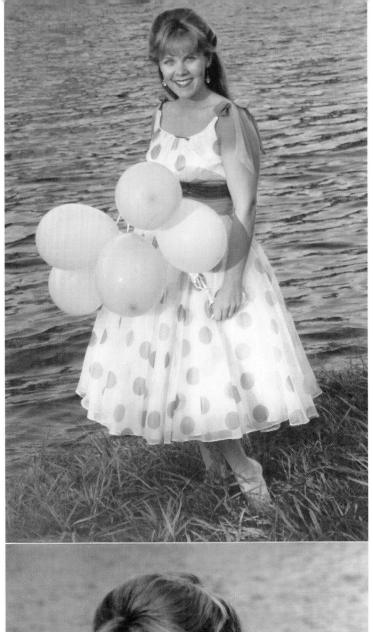

"San Francisco has a bank entirely managed by girls. The janitor is the only male employee...it is the Chinatown branch of the Bank of America...this is the first all-girl bank I've heard of. Have you heard of others?"
- Today's Woman, January 1951.

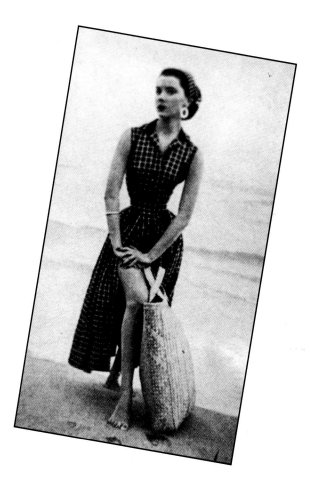

This Carolyn Schnurer red plaid playsuit, comprised of a bodice with attached shorts and a separate long skirt, was cover news for the June 1955 issue of *Charm*, and was designed by Carolyn Schnurer. (See the ready-to-wear designer list for more information on this playsuit.)

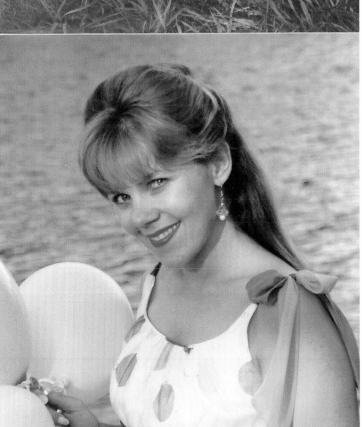

This unusual and absolutely fifties chiffon party dress features multi-colored chiffon ties at the shoulder and waist, and is printed with vari-colored balloons. *Courtesy of The Very Little Theatre.*

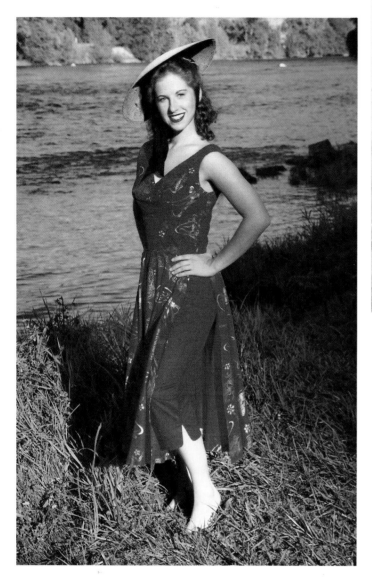

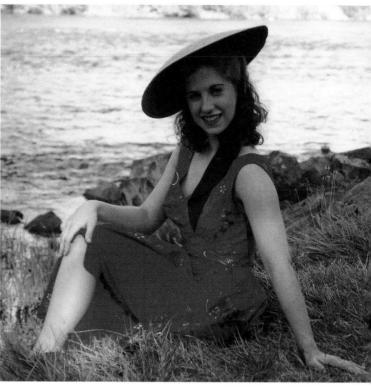

A fabulous play suit of gold-shot cotton. The complete dress is worn over separate Capri pants. *Courtesy of Persona Vintage Clothing.*

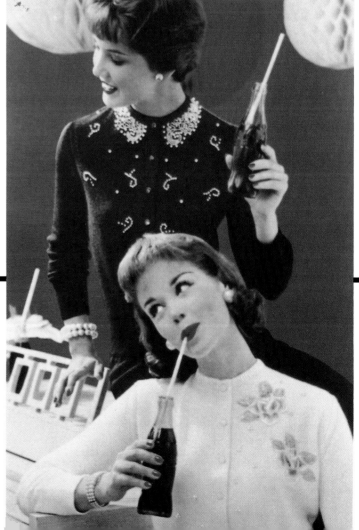

From the late 1950s, a Mazet ad featuring typical decorative sweaters for about $6.

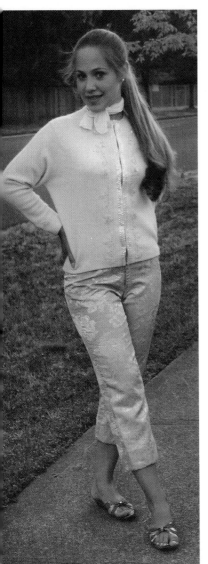

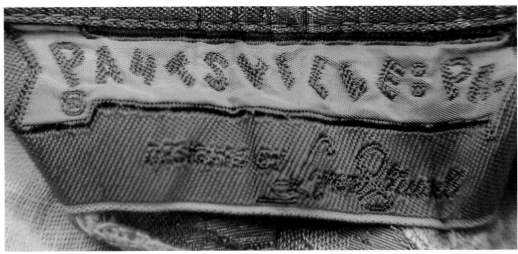

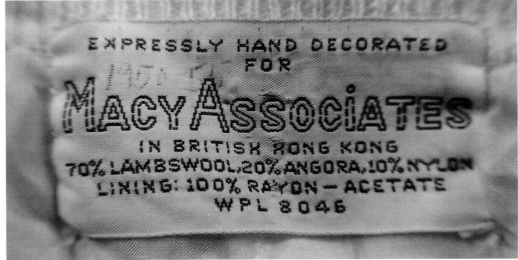

Perhaps in hopes of making pants more feminine, they were often elaborate. These peddle pushers are a classic example, made of gold-metallic shot brocade. Their label reads: "Pantsville: Pa. Designed by Lynn Stuart." The lambswool, angora, and nylon sweater is another fifties classic, featuring delicate white beading and a front hook and eye closure. It has a Macy's label but was hand beaded in Hong Kong. *Courtesy of The Very Little Theatre.*

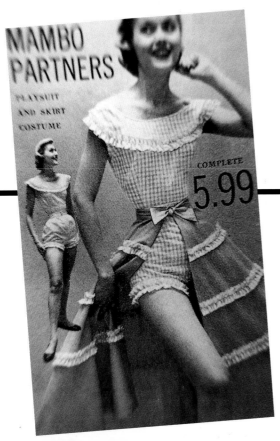

A 1955 ad by Paris for a gingham romper suit of attached bodice and shorts, with a separate tie-on overskirt in solid cotton. Available in baby blue or pink, the ensemble was sold for $5.99.

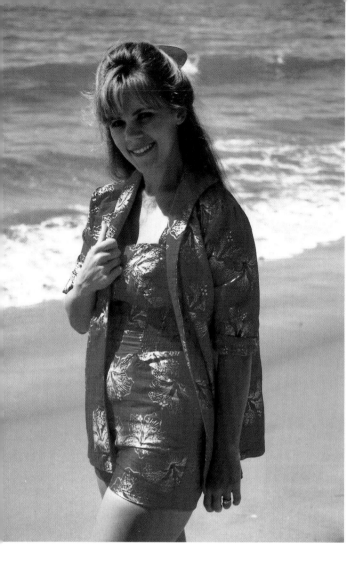

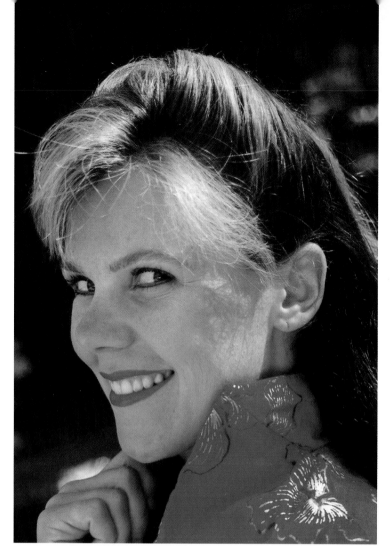

A bathing suit ideal for lounging. Made of 100% cotton, suits like these could be swum in, but would look untidy and wrinkled unless removed almost immediately after taking a dip. The bodice is boned and smocked, and the entire suit is fully lined in muslin, with elasticized bloomers beneath the outer, slim and fitted skirt. The matching overblouse features flexible collar steels, so that the chic woman could wear her collar sticking straight up.

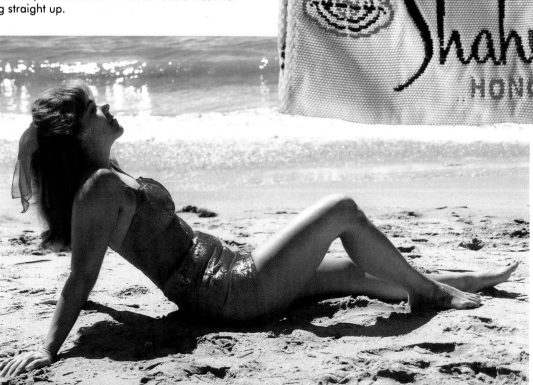

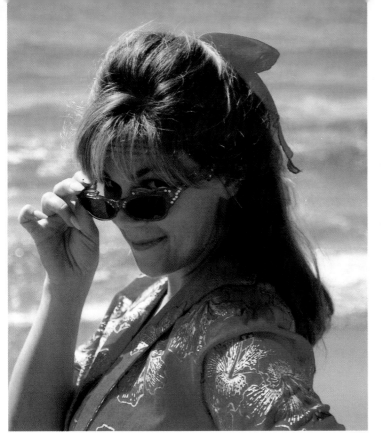

Though many fun and decorative plastic sunglasses were worn in the 1950s, they are difficult to find today. This pair is of blue plastic with both the cat's eye look and a wave design punctuated by silver stars. It is marked "Italy."

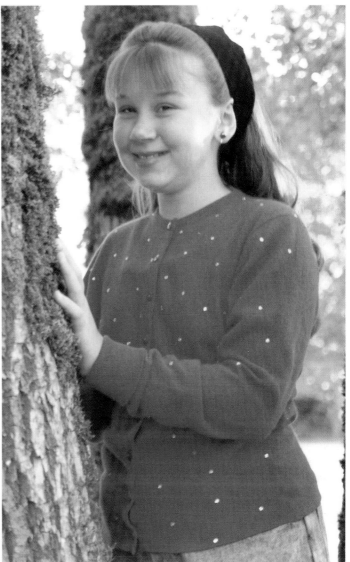

A coveted angora sweater, embellished with tiny rhinestones.

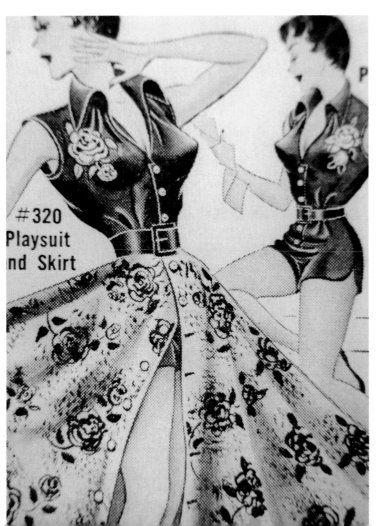

#320
Playsuit
nd Skirt

Fredrick's of Hollywood offered this more mature playsuit, also in 1955. Dubbed "Summer Secret," it consisted of a one piece shorts suit of cotton under a flowing skirt and patent belt. In "orange ice, purple, or sky blue," it sold for $11.98.

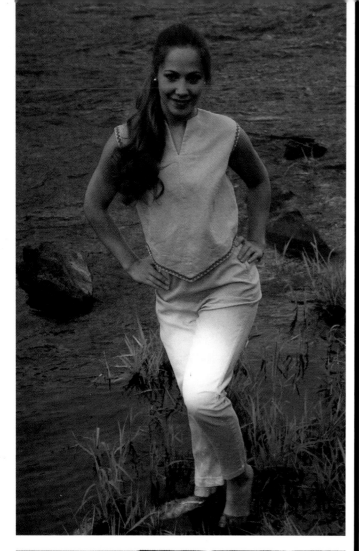

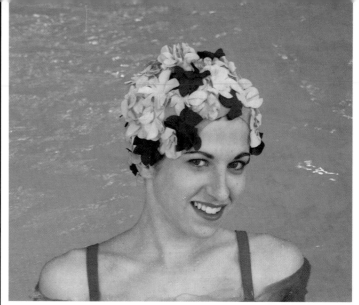

A delightful flowered bathing cap, dating to the late 1950s. *Courtesy of Flossy McGrew's.*

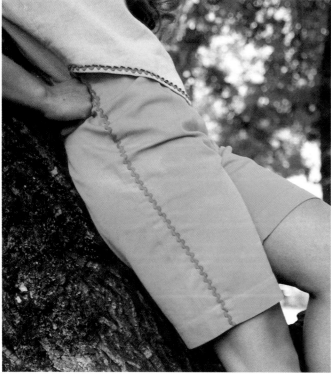

An unusual threesome: A pink corduroy blouse trimmed with blue rickrack, which may be worn with either matching corduroy Capris, or contrasting blue corduroy shorts. *Courtesy of Persona Vintage Clothing.*

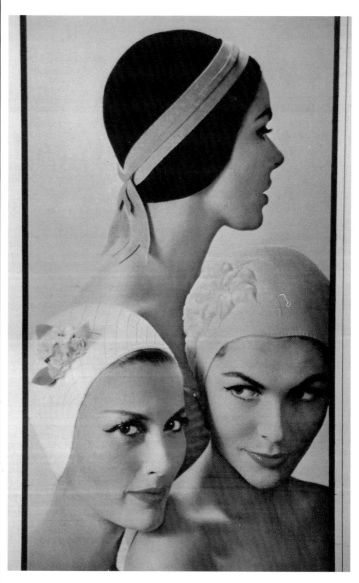

Bathing caps became aesthetic in the 1950s, and would continue to steal the beach scene in the 1960s. These three rubber caps, from a 1957 U.S. Swim Caps ad, show fifties bathing caps at their most artful.

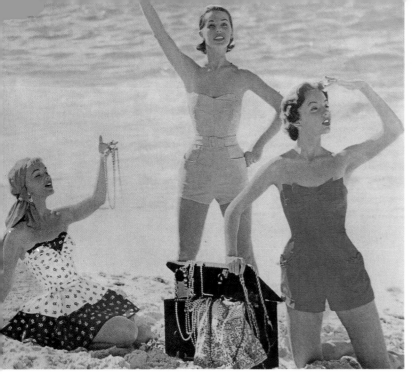

From a 1955 Brilliant Sportswear ad, these bathing suits show the range of fifties bathing suits—from tailored and trim, to flowing and ultra-feminine.

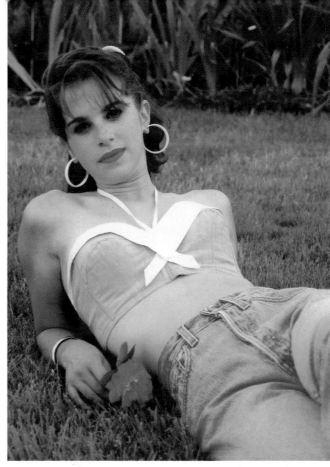

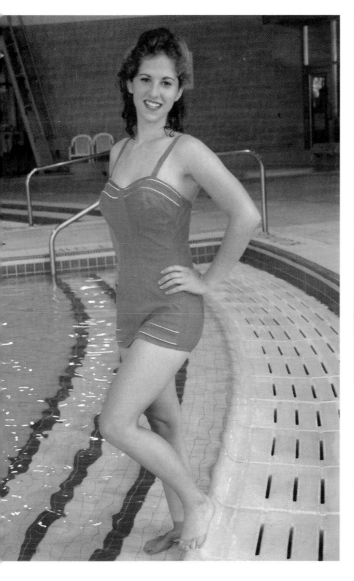

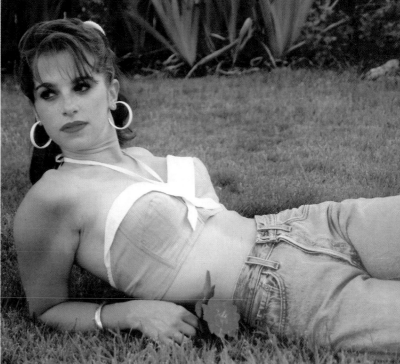

Of denim and a white (almost plastic-like) man-made material, this halter top is well boned for a "bullet" effect.

For those who preferred to be modest at the pool-side, a one-piece suit like this one by Catalina proved both flattering and comfortable. *Courtesy of Flossy McGrew's.*

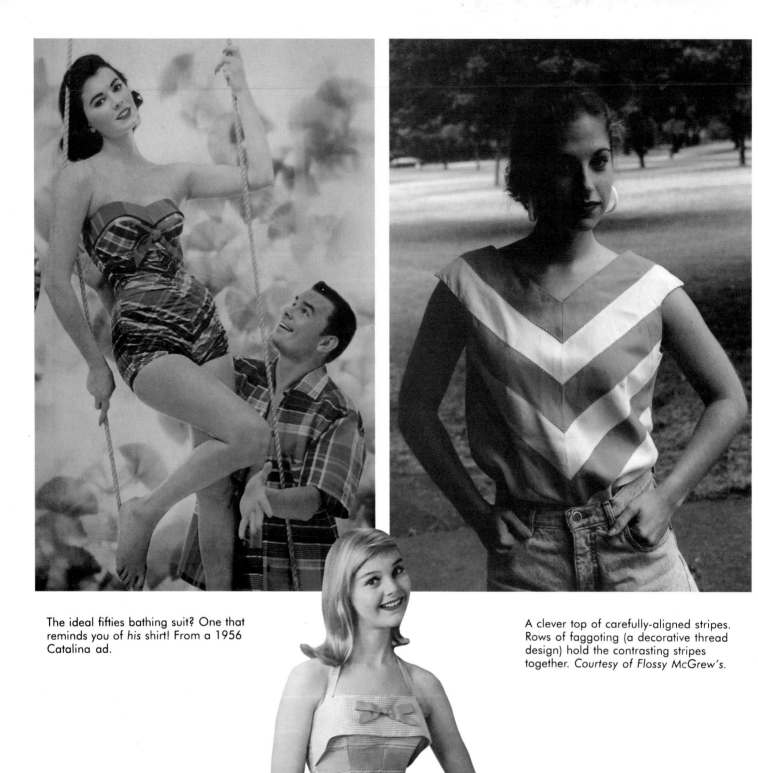

The ideal fifties bathing suit? One that reminds you of *his* shirt! From a 1956 Catalina ad.

A clever top of carefully-aligned stripes. Rows of faggoting (a decorative thread design) hold the contrasting stripes together. *Courtesy of Flossy McGrew's.*

A perfectly uncomfortable-looking bathing suit from a 1957 Maurice Handler ad.

maurice handler *Original*

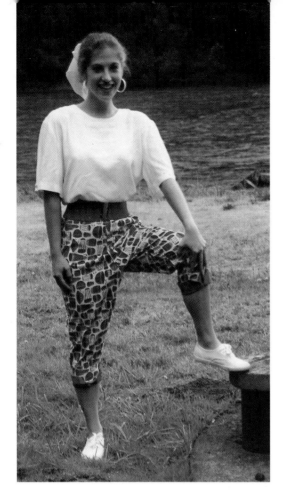

Colorful and playful peddle pushers
with a wide elasticized belt. *Courtesy of
Flossy McGrew's.*

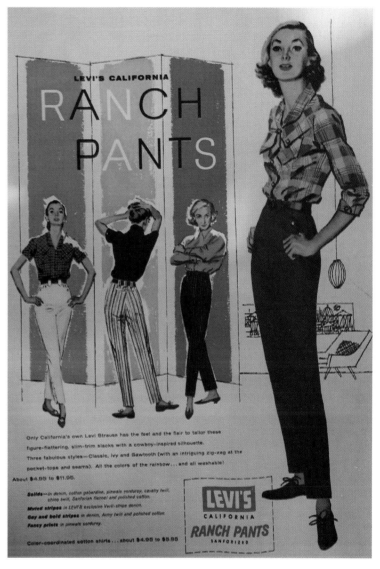

Levi's called their women's jeans "ranch pants"—a name
originating in the 1940s when women often had to wear
eminently practical clothing. These jeans—from a 1956 ad—
ranged in price from $4.95 to $11.95.

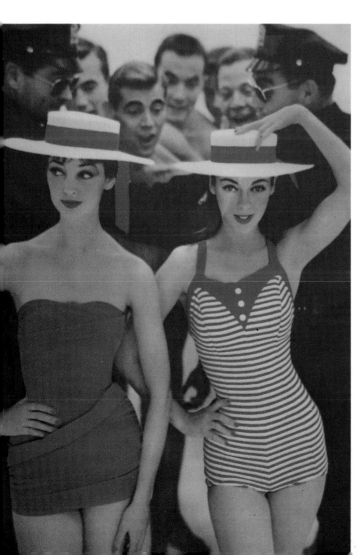

Cole of California made their idea of
the reaction a good bathing suit should
have very clear in a 1957 ad in
Seventeen.

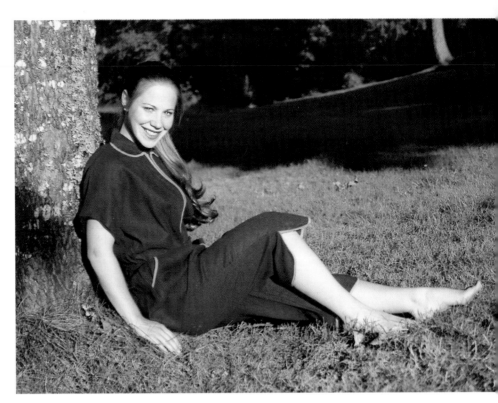

An unusual play suit of denim with bright turquoise piping trim. *Courtesy of Persona Vintage Clothing.*

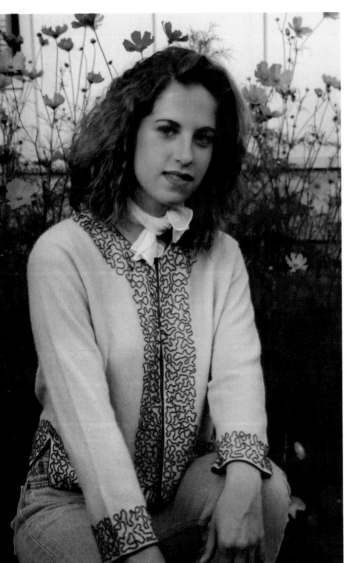

"Sew a week-end wardrobe for $7.50. Sewing gets easier all the time. This four-piece costume, for example, is made from a pattern with directions printed right on it. The box-jacket suit, weskit and shorts are actually two patterns but are priced as one...The total cost, including buttons and zippers: $7.50."
- *1950 pattern by Butterick.*

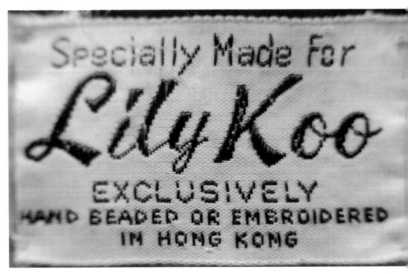

An angora and rabbit sweater with decorative beading. Like many beaded items of the era, it was created in Hong Kong. *Courtesy of The Very Little Theatre.*

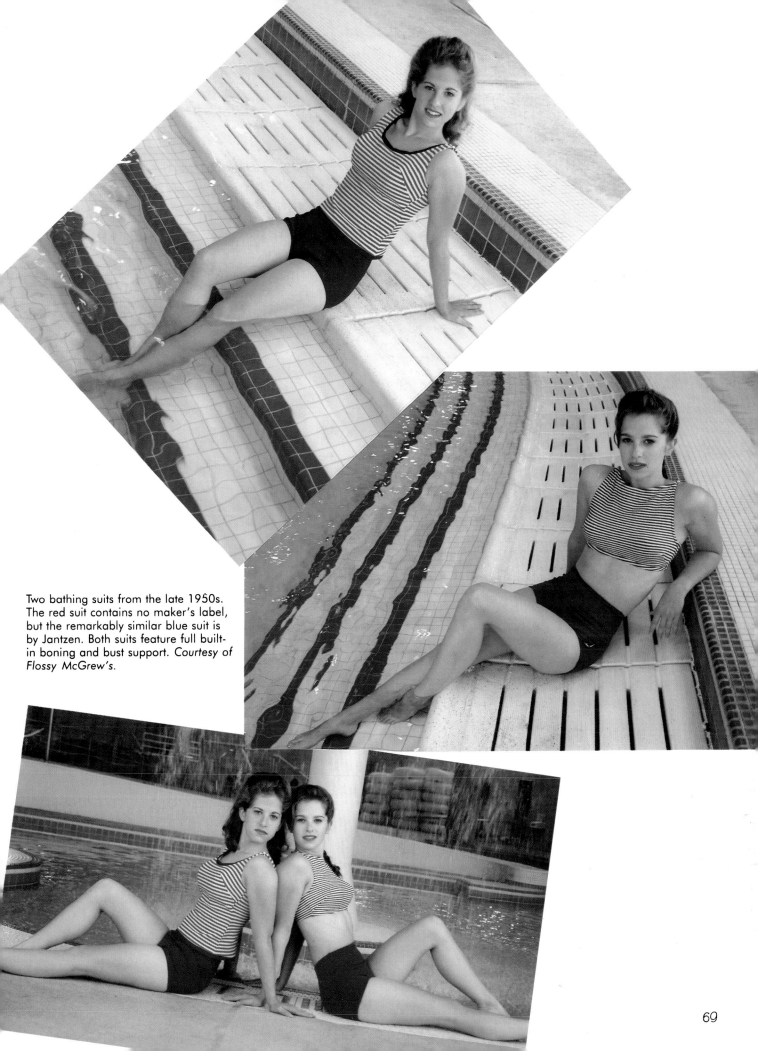

Two bathing suits from the late 1950s. The red suit contains no maker's label, but the remarkably similar blue suit is by Jantzen. Both suits feature full built-in boning and bust support. *Courtesy of Flossy McGrew's.*

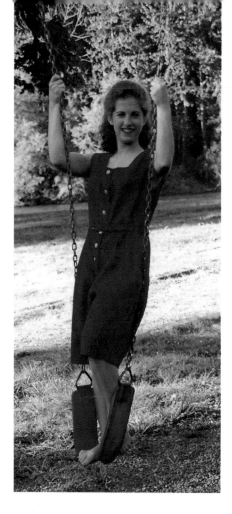

A simple playsuit of denim with turquoise plastic buttons. *Courtesy of Persona Vintage Clothing.*

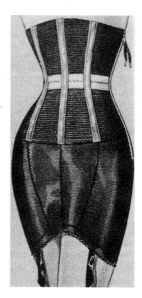

A corset, advertised in 1960.

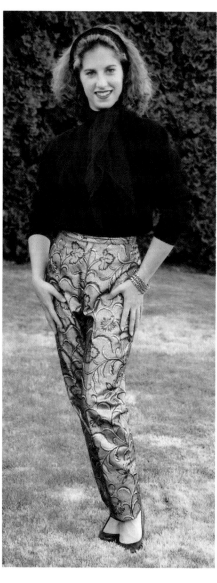

Metallic gold and black slacks by Pantsville.

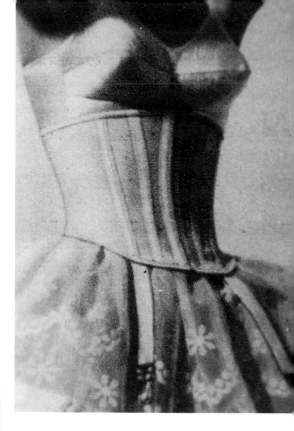

A corset with attached garters, by Kleinert's.

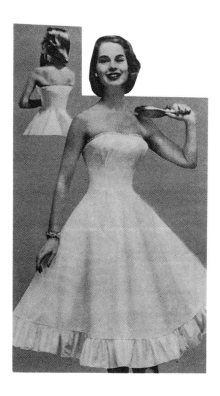

Advertised in 1957, one-piece undergarments like this one (which includes a bra and crinoline) were popular during the 1950s.

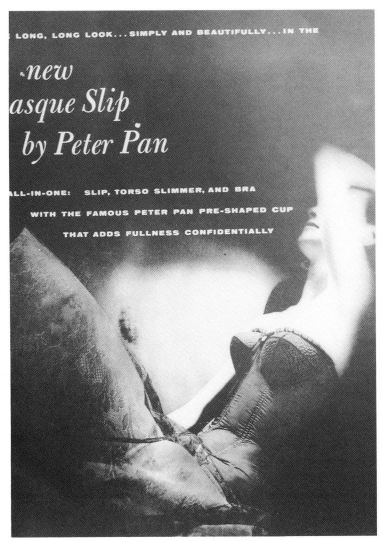

LONG, LONG LOOK... SIMPLY AND BEAUTIFULLY... IN THE

new
asque Slip
by Peter Pan

ALL-IN-ONE: SLIP, TORSO SLIMMER, AND BRA

WITH THE FAMOUS PETER PAN PRE-SHAPED CUP

THAT ADDS FULLNESS CONFIDENTIALLY

Another all-in-one, this one advertised by Peter Pan in 1953. The "Basque Slip" includes corset, bra, and crinoline.

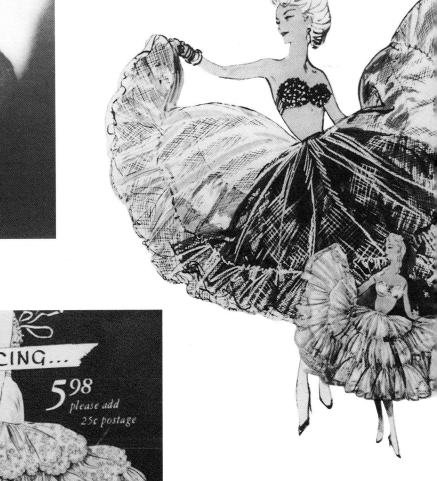

Advertised in a 1957 issue of *Seventeen*, two types of special-occasion crinolines.

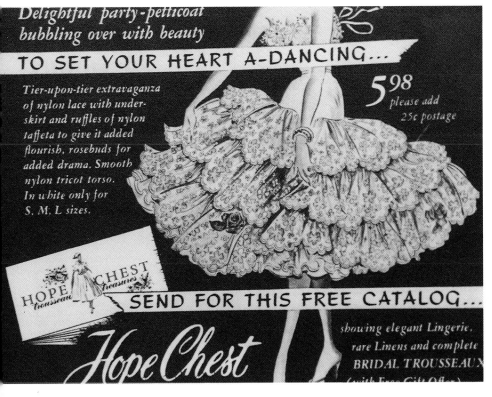

Delightful party-petticoat bubbling over with beauty

TO SET YOUR HEART A-DANCING...

Tier-upon-tier extravaganza of nylon lace with under-skirt and ruffles of nylon taffeta to give it added flourish, rosebuds for added drama. Smooth nylon tricot torso. In white only for S, M, L sizes.

5⁹⁸ please add 25c postage

HOPE CHEST *treasures*

SEND FOR THIS FREE CATALOG...

Hope Chest

showing elegant Lingerie, rare Linens and complete BRIDAL TROUSSEAUX

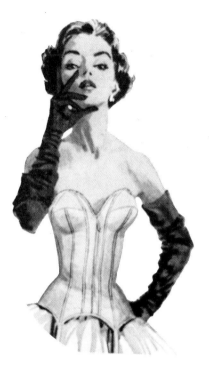

From a 1955 ad, a typical fifties-style corset.

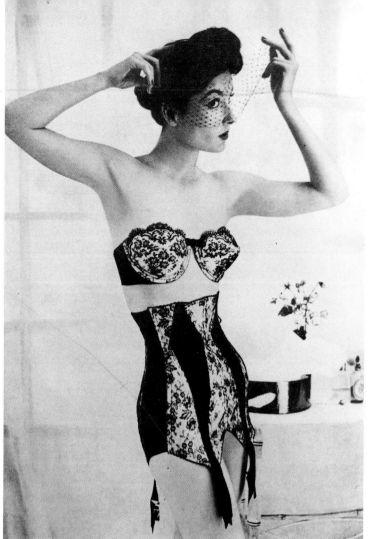

"The Witching Power," this 1952 Warner's ad headlined. Of Chantilly lace and powernet, the girdle nips in the waist and holds up stockings, while the matching bra is in the "new" boned bandeaux strapless style. The pair sold for $35.

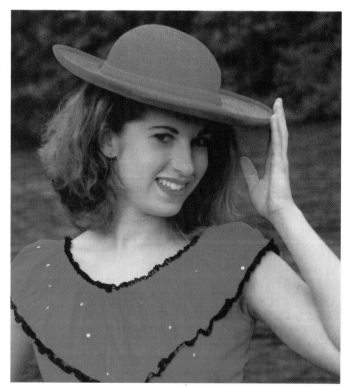

This simple straw hat is typical of those worn throughout the fifties and early sixties. *Courtesy of Flossy McGrew's.*

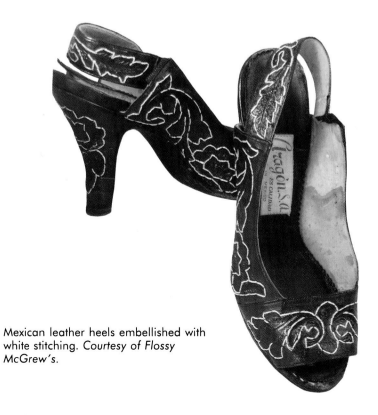

Mexican leather heels embellished with white stitching. *Courtesy of Flossy McGrew's.*

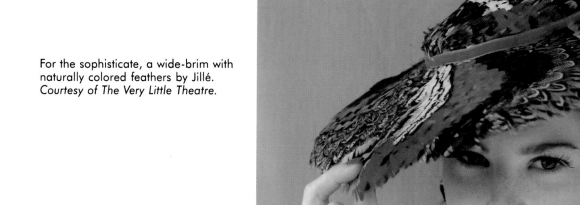

For the sophisticate, a wide-brim with naturally colored feathers by Jillé. *Courtesy of The Very Little Theatre.*

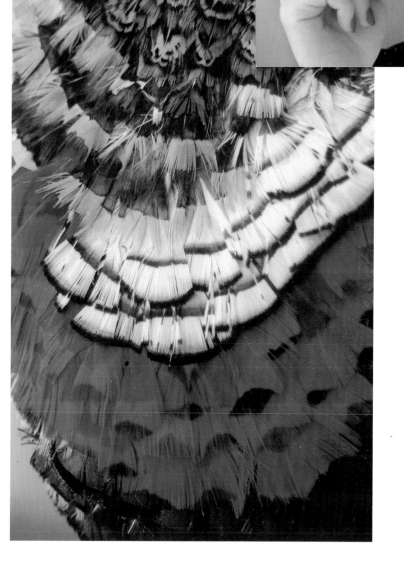

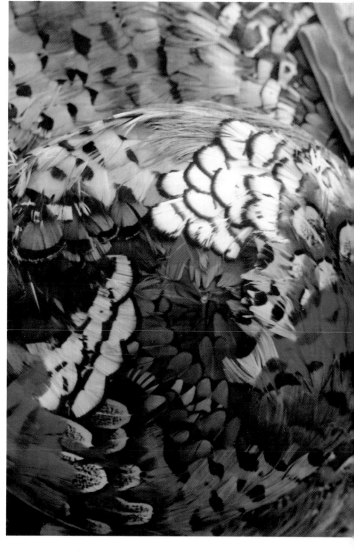

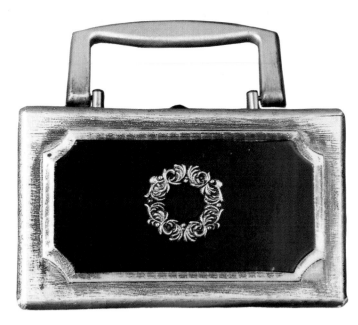

A wooden box purse trimmed with gold leaf. *Courtesy of The Very Little Theatre.*

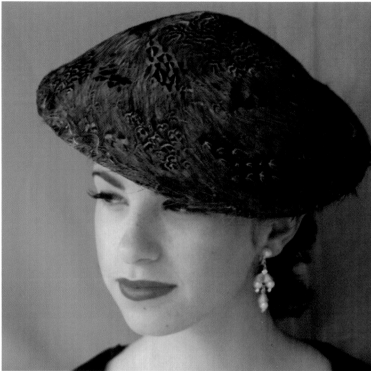

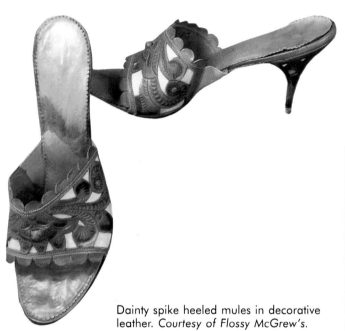

Dainty spike heeled mules in decorative leather. *Courtesy of Flossy McGrew's.*

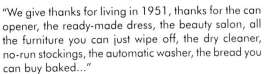
"We give thanks for living in 1951, thanks for the can opener, the ready-made dress, the beauty salon, all the furniture you can just wipe off, the dry cleaner, no-run stockings, the automatic washer, the bread you can buy baked..."
- *Today's Woman*, January 1951.

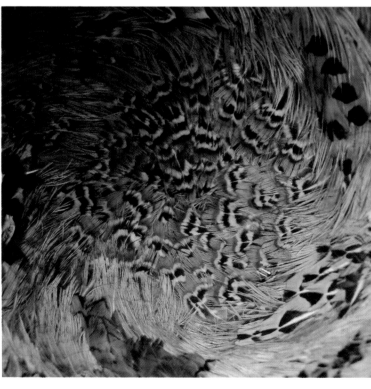

A classy feather hat labeled: "Leslie James, California." *Courtesy of The Very Little Theatre.*

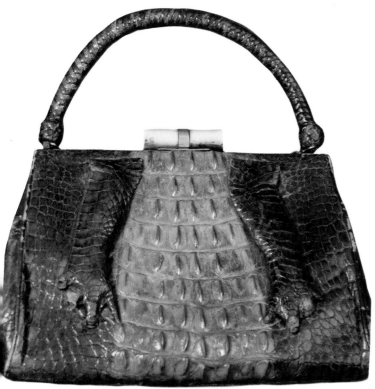

An alligator clutch with hints as to its origin. *Courtesy of Flossy McGrew's.*

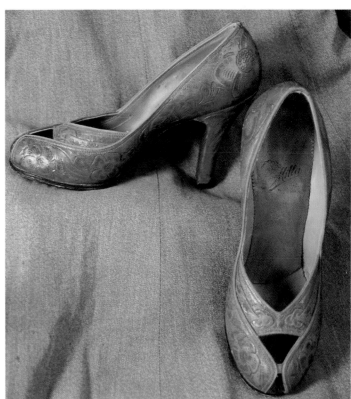

Heels of carved leather. *Courtesy of Flossy McGrew's.*

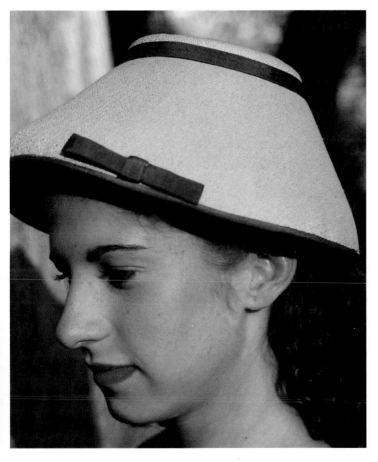

A "flower pot" hat from the fifties. Courtesy of *Flossy McGrew's.*

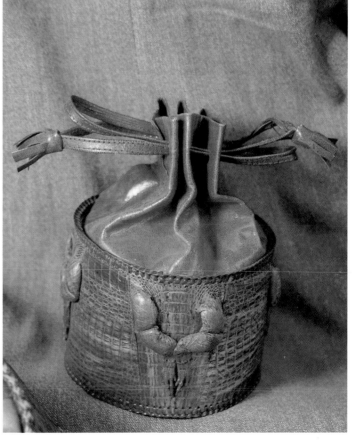

A small, round alligator bag made in Columbia and featuring four set of picturesque feet. Courtesy of *Flossy McGrew's.*

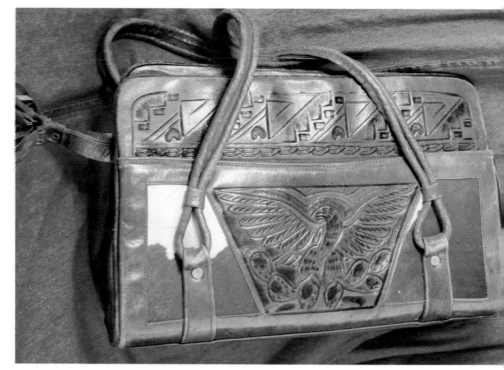

A rustic Western handbag of carved leather and cowhide. *Courtesy of Flossy McGrew's.*

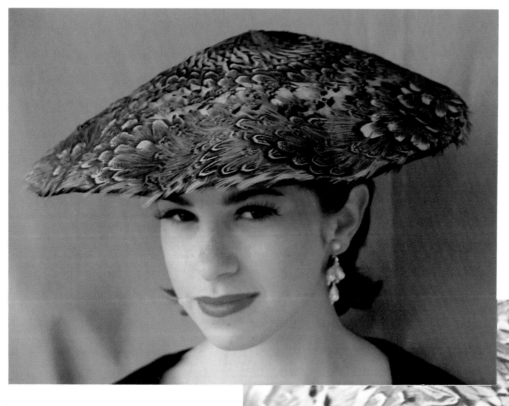

Labeled "Urbiet Orbi," this hat shows strong Oriental influence. *Courtesy of The Very Little Theatre.*

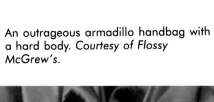

An outrageous armadillo handbag with a hard body. *Courtesy of Flossy McGrew's.*

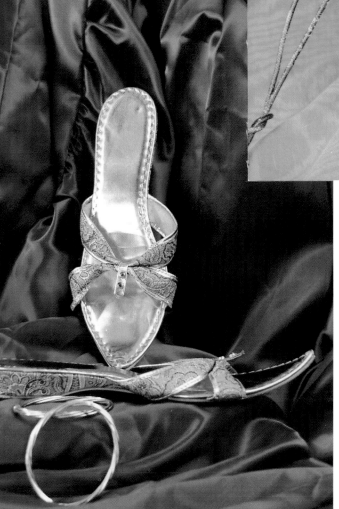

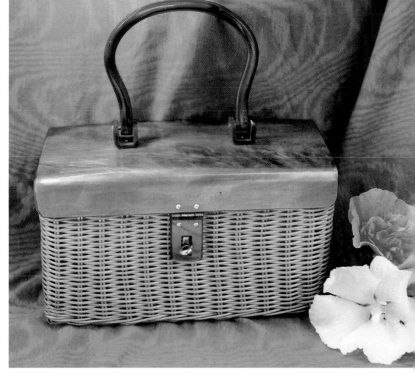

Middle-East inspired sandals with brocade straps tied together with pseudo-emeralds. *Courtesy of The Very Little Theatre.*

A wicker and Lucite handbag. *Courtesy of Persona Vintage Clothing.*

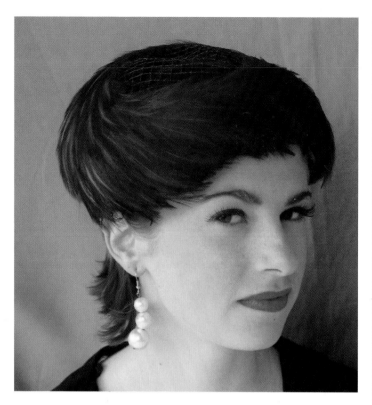

Though typically fifties in its small size and ever-so-common style, this hat commands attention with its brilliant blue feathers. *Courtesy of The Very Little Theatre.*

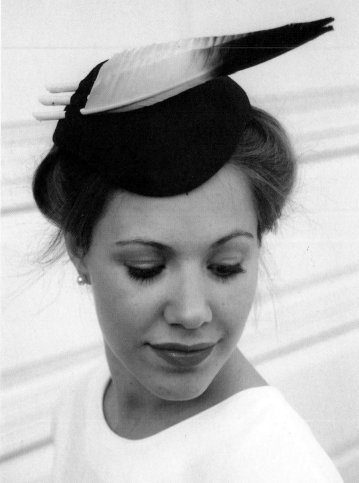

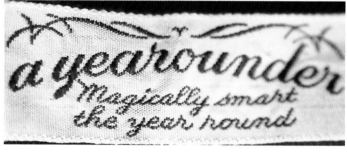

A tailored "Yearounder" felt hat c. 1949, punctuated with three feathers, to be worn with a business suit. *Courtesy of The Very Little Theatre.*

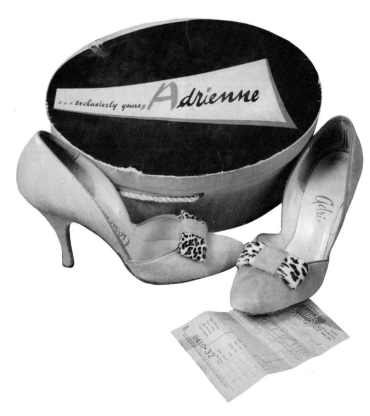

Goat hair heels in their original box and with their original sales receipt. *Courtesy of Flossy McGrew's.*

"Practicality...fashion's new emphasis. The wonders of man-made fibers woven into fabrics so heavenly to touch...so luxurious to wear...who could guess their astonishing practicality! Here, a go-everywhere suit...a bright cocktail dress...made with 'Dacron'...to resist wrinkles...keep their pleats even in a sudden shower...shed many spots with soap and water...stay fresh and comfortable through says of wearing. You'll find a whole new way to look...a new way to live...in 'Dacron'...one of Du Pont's fibers for practical fashions."
- *DuPont ad, 1952.*

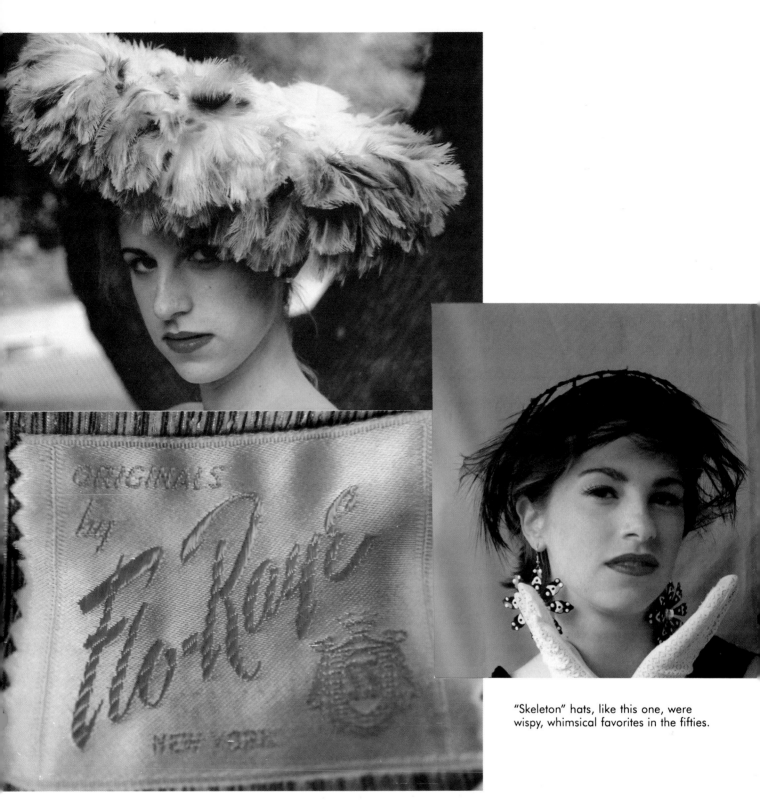

"Skeleton" hats, like this one, were wispy, whimsical favorites in the fifties.

A delectable ostrich feather hat by Flo-Raye. *Courtesy of Flossy McGrew's.*

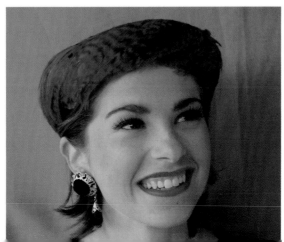

Small—but definitely not unobtrusive—this wildly colored hat is a "Valerie Modes." *Courtesy of The Very Little Theatre.*

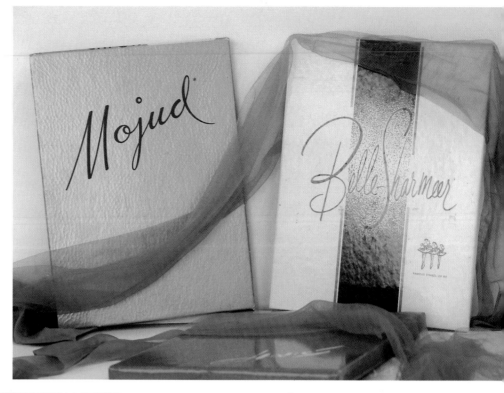

Stockings from the 1950s-60s are most collectible if in their original packaging (check to make certain the marking on the thigh matches the label on the box). Here, several seamed styles are shown from prevalent manufacturers.

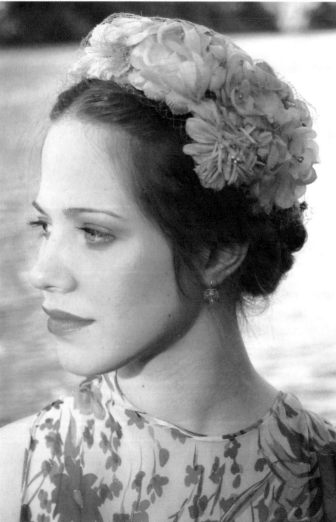

Lucite evening shoes with black design details. *Courtesy of Flossy McGrew's.*

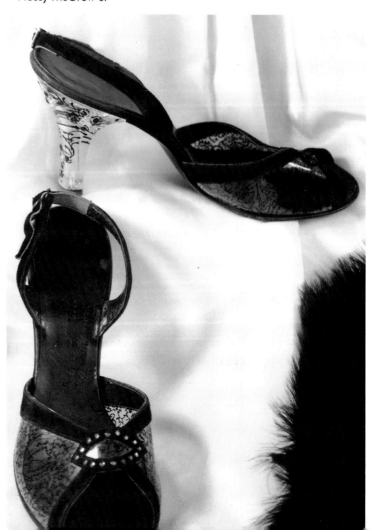

This dainty, flowered Valerie Modes hat is typical of the 1950s. *Courtesy of The Very Little Theatre.*

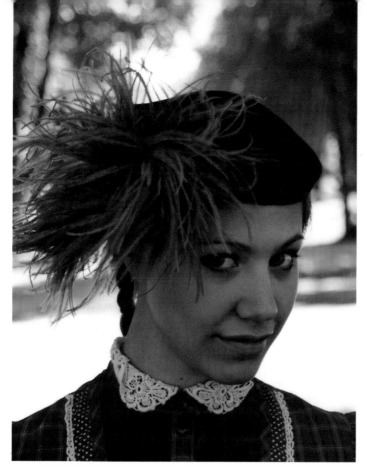

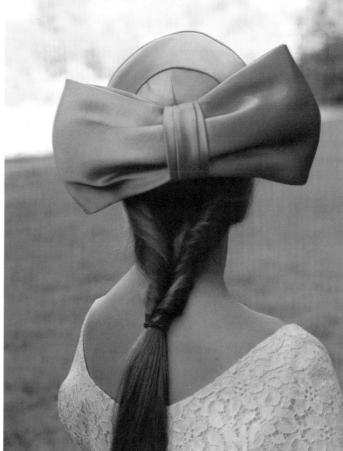

A fun fifties hat of felt with a large plume. The label reads: "Amy, New York." *Courtesy of The Very Little Theatre.*

A tiny straw hat from the 1950s, featuring ruching and three large rhinestones scattered around the brim. *Courtesy of The Very Little Theatre.*

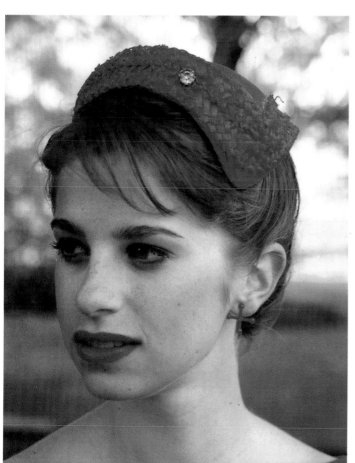

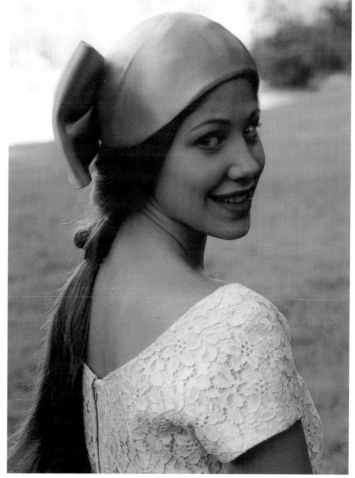

A silly satin hat, reminiscent of Minnie Mouse. *Courtesy of Flossy McGrew's.*

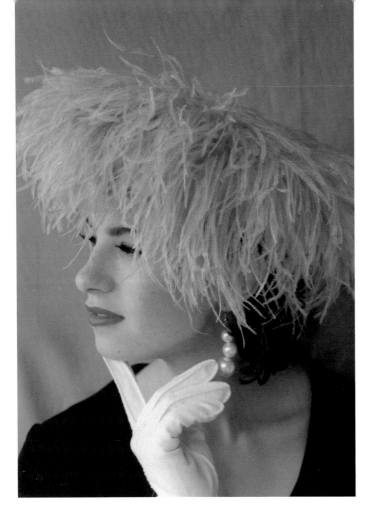

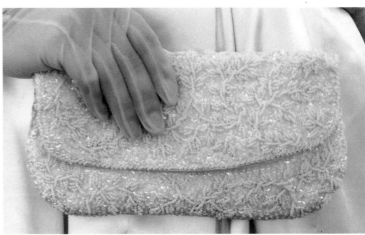

An all-over white glass beaded satin clutch evening purse from the fifties.

Dripping with pink marabou feathers, this darling is a "Deborah Exclusive." *Courtesy of The Very Little Theatre.*

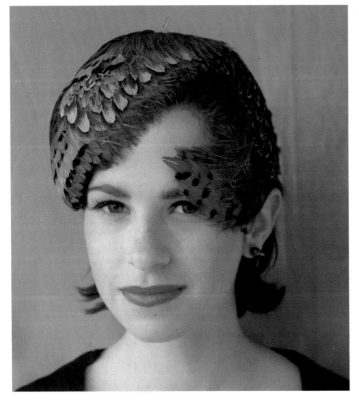

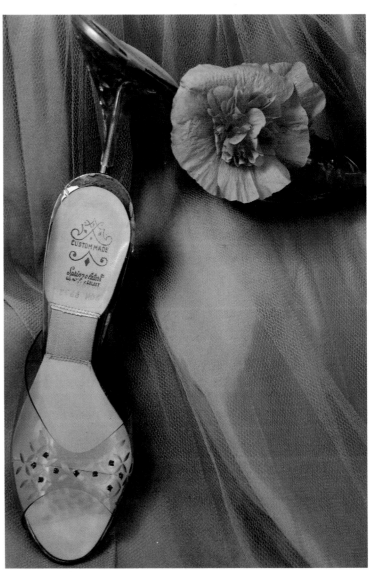

Some feather hats make no bones about their origin; this hat is cleverly shaped to suggest a bird-like formation, and even features a faux beak. *Courtesy of The Very Little Theatre.*

Lucite evening shoes from the late fifties or early sixties. *Courtesy of Flossy McGrew's.*

A beach purse of canvas. Decorated with faux sea shells and featuring a draw-string closure, it would hold little more than sunglasses, lotion, and perhaps a snack. *Courtesy of The Very Little Theatre.*

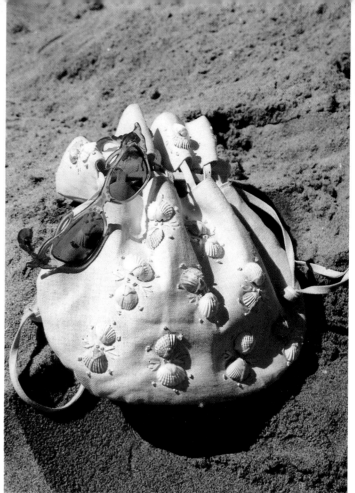

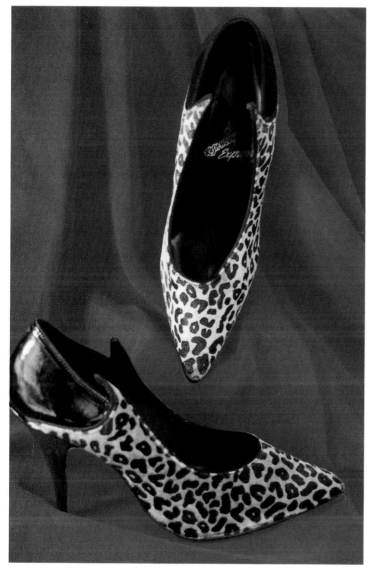

"Leopard skin" spike heels. *Courtesy of Flossy McGrew's.*

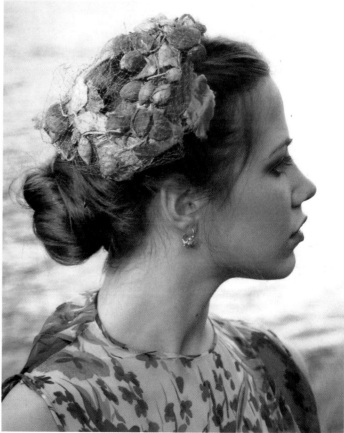

Made up of faux flowers encased in netting, this pillbox dates to the early sixties and carries a "Valerie Modes" label. *Courtesy of The Very Little Theatre.*

"I've always dated several boys at a time—I think that's the only way to find the right husband."
- *Miss America 1958 in the November 1957 issue of Seventeen.*

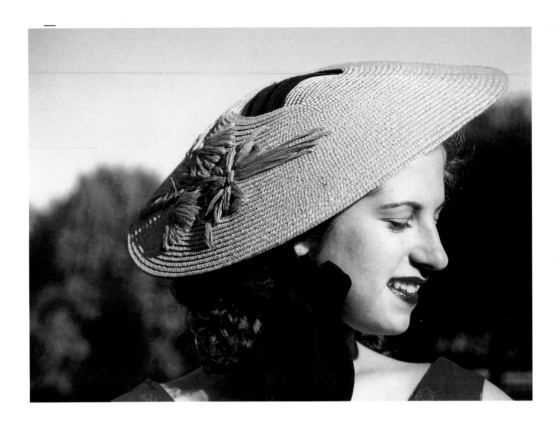

An Orient-inspired straw hat decorated with dyed straw
threaded into flower shapes. The ties are of rayon.

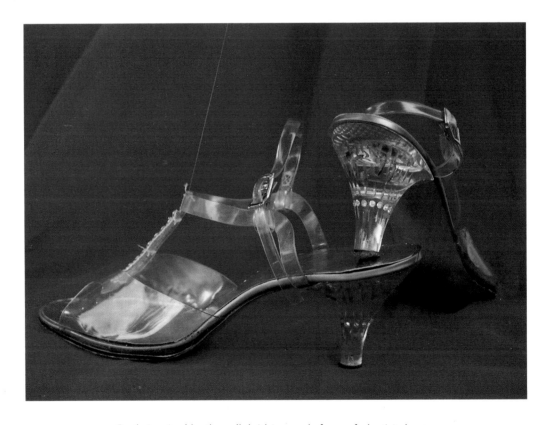

Partly inspired by the celluloid (an early form of plastic) shoes
of W.W.II and partly inspired by fabled Cinderella's glass
slippers, Lucite evening shoes like these were popular throughout the 1950s and early 1960s. These have a Good Housekeeping Seal of Approval and are made by Dream Step
Originals. *Courtesy of The Very Little Theatre.*

The 1960s

Fashion Goes Public

By 1966, the ready-to-wear industry accounted for $14,000,000,000 of business, and couture designer business made up only 12% of all dresses sold in the United States. Adding power behind them, the five biggest ready-to-wear manufacturers went public: Jonathan Logan, Bobbie Brooks, Russ Togs, Puritan, and Leslie Fay. Lumped together, these companies newly on the stock market exchange produced over 70,000,000 garments, which were then sold through some 30,000 retail stores. Bobbie Brooks—the first to appear on the stock exchange—was about as far from couture as possible. Instead of having designers hand down new styles from on high, the company formed a panel of 600 young women to judge their clothing. Majority ruled in what actually became available in the stores. From these publicly-owned ready-to-wear companies, most of the clothing sold was priced for the consumer at about $12-$30 a piece.

To add to these exciting new innovations in the garment industry, mail-order sales continued to rise as well. Smaller companies had found success selling specific garments through ads in the back of fashion magazines since the 19th century, but companies like Sears, Roebuck, & Company and Montgomery Ward had distributed mail order catalogs since the 1880s with incredible success. In the 1960s J.C. Penny was added to this list. Though this company had successfully operated retail stores since 1902, it wasn't until 1966 that they produced their first mail order catalog—and an innovative and modern catalog it was, featuring fashions from Paris, London, and Madrid photographed in famous spots from all three cities. Classy as this might sound, prices were moderate; a dress for $9, a coat for $16—though more expensive items (such as a coat from Madrid for $40) were also available. The same year they produced their first catalog, *Women's Wear Daily* reported that 7% of all coats and 6% of all non-knitted dresses sold in the United States were purchased from J.C. Penny. By 1967, Penny's, Sears, and Montgomery Ward combined accounted for about $6,000,000,000 of all national retail sales.

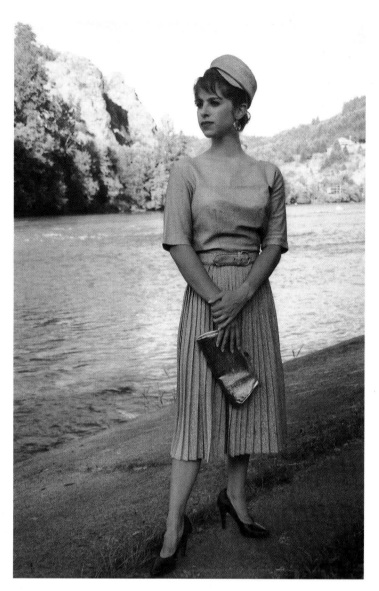

This all-metallic early sixties ensemble features a blouse, pleated skirt, and matching belt with the popular Koret of California label. *Courtesy of The Very Little Theatre.*

As the ready-to-wear industry's success skyrocketed, the cost of dressing plummeted. In 1967, manufacturers of moderate to inexpensive garments claimed that for several years 40% of all dresses sold (about 110,000,000 dresses total) were $5.98 or less, and that "all but 12% of all dresses sold for less than $25"—that's 233,000,000 dresses.

In 1967, fashion writer Jessica Daves literally wrote the book on the ready-to-wear industry. In awe, she titled the book appropriately—*The Ready-To-Wear Miracle*—and her text overflows with wonder at the ease and cheapness to consumers the new industry provided. She quotes a fictional—though realistic—conversation:

"Lady, to lady magazine editor, at dinner party: 'Do you see this dress! Your September issue came yesterday, the dress was right on page ninety-nine, clear as Baccarat crystal. It said—you said in the

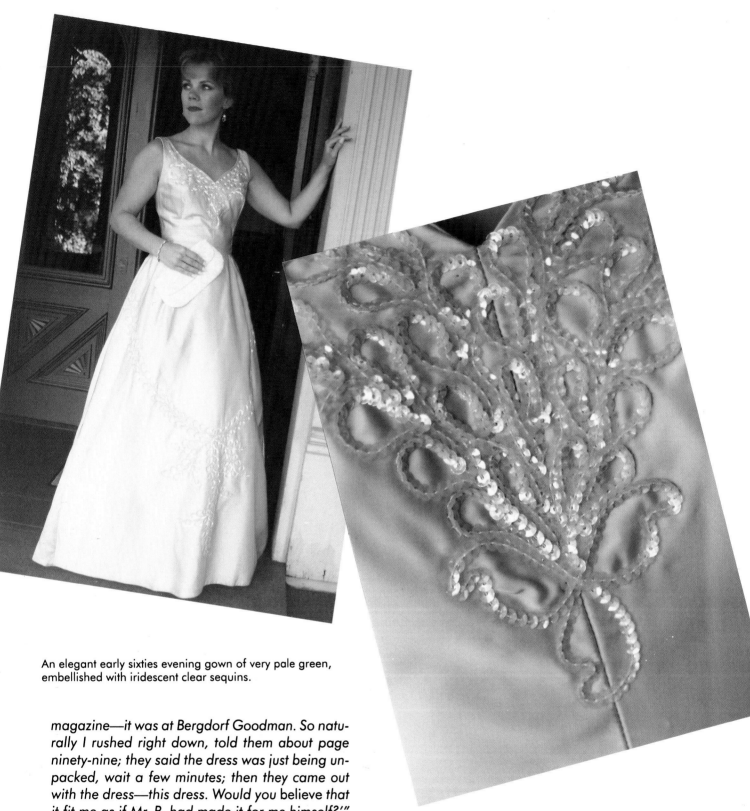

An elegant early sixties evening gown of very pale green, embellished with iridescent clear sequins.

magazine—it was at Bergdorf Goodman. So naturally I rushed right down, told them about page ninety-nine; they said the dress was just being unpacked, wait a few minutes; then they came out with the dress—this dress. Would you believe that it fit me as if Mr. B. had made it for me himself?'"

Taking us to 463 Seventh Avenue, New York City, where a great many manufacturers of inexpensive women's garments resided, Daves also offers an unprecedented look into just how the ready-to-wear industry functioned technically during the sixties:

"*In the big, quiet, cutting room just inside the door, the pattern makers are turning the dress designer's ideas into oddly shaped pieces of cardboard, as many as sixteen pieces for one dress. At the back of the room, working at a table that looks almost half a block long, a man is bending over this series of little shaped pieces of cardboard, fitting them as neatly as possible into the forty-five-inch-wide material stretched on the table. He moves them around until magically there seems to be enough space between only for the blade of a thin knife; having done that, he goes from pattern piece to pattern piece, punching holes in certain* strategic spots. On an adjoining table a cutter works on a similar, pattern-covered length of cloth. The length of cloth turns out to be 400 layers of cloth, and on the top layer the pattern pieces are placed exactly according to the careful plotting on the neighboring table. The electrically driven knife goes through the 400 layers as cleanly as the Cordless Cutter goes through cheese. Once the pieces are cut, tiny holes are punched in what seemed to be random markings of the magician who had fitted the pattern to the cloth on the other table. These are the guidelines for the workers who presently take over the patterns. Lying on the table is a six-handled, flat, small metal machine about a foot square: the size grader. This is a vital part of the cutting, making it possible to change the measurements from size eight to size sixteen, accurately, and to come out with the same dress, ready for the machines. The sewing is done in another building on West 23rd Street...

"Besides the markers and cutters, more than 100 girls work there at the sewing machines. Soft music is played most of the time, not persistent and not too loud, just a pleasant background...Even in this inexpensive house, many of these workers make the complete dress except for the finishing [for example, the fastenings]...These costumes...are more complicated than a shift [dress], which, with lining, consists of about sixteen separate pieces and is made by the section method...Individual girls make these individual parts of the dress, and they are then put together by other workers."

"How much [fabric] do they buy at one time?" Daves questioned further. "Of one fabric? 'Oh, about twenty thousand yards to start...' (Twenty thousand yards is a little more than eleven and one-third miles, or about a quarter-mile shorter than Manhattan island.)" The author, and every woman who cherished her ability to purchase attractive clothing inexpensively and easily, was dazzled.

Power In Print

Of course, no ready-to-wear manufacturer or designer could be successful without women who needed inexpensive, fashionable clothing, and—significantly—fashion magazines who would let women everywhere know about them. One manufacturer was so keenly aware of this that in 1960, its president wrote to *Vogue*:

"Referring to the cotton-knit situation which has been the bulwark of our operation since 1954, I would like you to know that we were virtually pushed into this business by your Mrs. McManus [fashion editor]. In February of 1954 we were asked [by Mrs. McManus] to style a T-shirt dress [for the youth section]...As I recall, I had never heard of a T-shirt dress before that time but we and the industry have heard a great deal about them since..."

The power of the fashion magazine was not to be ignored! Though in the 19th century, such magazines were used by designers and manufacturers to help peddle their creations and—even in the 20th century—the magazine itself did little but parrot what designers told them was fashionable and correct, by the 1950s-

Subtleties in length and construction (including no attached crinoline or linings to make the skirt stand out fuller) date this chiffon print dress to the sixties. *Courtesy of The Very Little Theatre.*

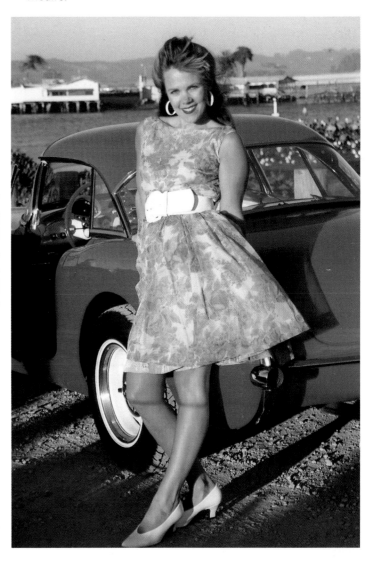

60s, the fashion magazine was its own force to be reckoned with. No designer or manufacturer could afford to not cater to the top magazines. Upon having a coat featured on the cover of *Mademoiselle*, for example, one manufacturer sold 4,500 copies of the same coat from 158 stores across the United States. Similarly, *Glamour* featured a sweater on their August 1964 cover and 18,000 copies of that sweater were reported sold shortly after. On April 1, 1966, *Vogue* featured a green jersey dress, and by July 1, 25,000 had been sold. And proving the power of the new teenage market, after *Seventeen* featured one bathing suit in their June 1965 issue, 50,000 were sold across the United States.

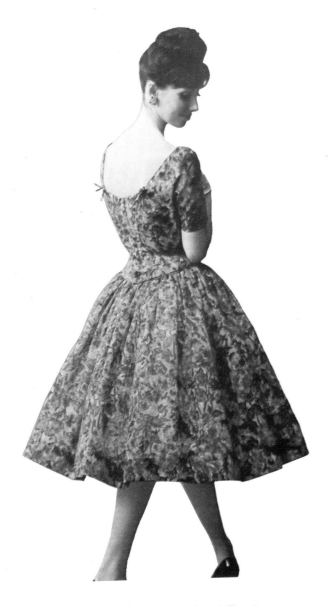

A 1960 ad featuring the ever-popular chiffon dress.

Slight Revisions & New Quests

Many of the neo-Victorian styles of the late fifties lingered in the 1960s; dresses with tight bodices and full skirts remained popular—though they tended to have shorter skirts and be less "frilly." Trapeze (now often called "tent") dresses, too, were as comfortable as ever, and many women clung to them. *Mademoiselle* was still praising the tent as late as 1967: "Ladies! Your attention pu-leaze!" the editors cried like circus barkers. "Fork over, and you've a tent you can live in. A tiny swirl of plaid voile...$16!" The empire waist, too, was cherished for its comfort, even if it tended to give women a "baby doll" look—or, if it had a gathered skirt, a pregnant appearance. The 1920s revival of tube-like dresses with lowered waistlines and pleated skirts also continued to find success, as did pleated skirts worn with hip-length blouses. Even *The New York Times* noted the 1920s fashion-revival in 1965: "The flapper's slip of a dress has proved as functional for the Frug as it was for the Charleston." In fact, though we tend to associate the sixties with hippies, it wasn't until the last few years of the 1960s that "radical rags" and the flower-child looks began having a strong influence on mainstream fashion; throughout most of the 1960s, women dressed in a fashion very similar to the previous decade.

Little was really new; most fashions were only revised versions of Dior's "New Look." Even the new shift dress was only a more shapely version of the sack, fitting softly over the bust, defining slightly the waist, and featuring a straight skirt—little different than the fifties chemise. In 1963, a trend for dresses with softly-shaped, blouse-like bodices began to emerge; sleeves were barely gathered into the shoulder, and were often gathered into wide wristbands. By evening, dresses were largely sleeveless, and often knee-length. "The newest aspect [in] formals," *McCall's Fashion Patterns* noted in 1960, "is the slender siren dress in clingy black or blazing glitter fabric...In brilliant contrast is the full-length full-fledged ball gown, making its street-length rivals of recent years seem somehow not quite dressed." The Chanel-style suit (in particular, the knitted suit) found continued success, and we might even imagine that some women discovered circa 1920s Chanel styles in their grandmother's closets, and adopted them for street wear; since Chanel hadn't revised her fashions much, the old Chanel would appear equally as up-to-date as the new Chanel—and in fact, many young women found twenties styles in thrift shops and put them to new use.

"About that favorite suit that jumps to mind at the idea of a date at the beach, make sure that it fits the occasion as well as yourself. If you can slip into it with a fair amount of ease, fine. If you have to struggle into it, and it needs perpetual adjusting, better wear something else, so that you feel natural and comfortable, which is a girl's nicest outdoor look."
-*Charm*, July 1959.

But if the fifties had been about firm foundations and structure, the sixties was about setting the body free from foundations and moving in on the natural human form. "I compromised when business partners were content for me to make only little empire dresses stiffened to hide a multitude of sins. I stopped compromising when I bought my own business and went 'soft,' moving in on the body and all its glory. I do not compromise any more," says Geoffrey Beane, one of the first coutures to begin this trend. In his own words, his goal as a designer is to "liberate the body while adorning it." Something that hadn't been done since the dress reform movements of the 1890s (when "freeing" the body meant trading in a long, ungainly corset for a shorter, non-boned body-binder). In keeping with this increasingly popular attitude, the T-shirt dress of the 1950s had become a staple of most every young woman's wardrobe—prompting manufacturers to expand their collections of knitted dresses; by 1967, knitted clothing accounted for over $2,000,000,000 of the money spent on fashions in the United States—twice as much as in 1954 when the T-shirt dress was introduced.

Perhaps this new quest for body freedom is what inspired the mini-skirt. First appearing in 1961 on some very brave (some might say brash) young women, the look caught *Life* magazine's eye, prompting a feature titled: "American Current Teenage Fad—the Short Skirt." Still only three or four inches above the knee, the short skirt was anything but a fad—and by 1965, mid-thigh skirts were worn by young women everywhere, prompting both shock and humor. Shock because no woman had ever worn skirts so short in public—ever, in all of history. And humor because progress in stockings was noticeably behind progress in skirts; garters were still necessary to hold stockings up, and, when worn with mini-skirts, these often revealed themselves with the slightest move. To avoid being humorous (which, after all, was not the point), many young women went bare-legged, like their flapper grandmothers. (Later in the 1960s, somebody figured out that the tights ballet dancers had been wearing for decades worked just as well for street-wear, and young women in mini-skirts soon happily adopted them. Shortly after, panty-hose appeared.)

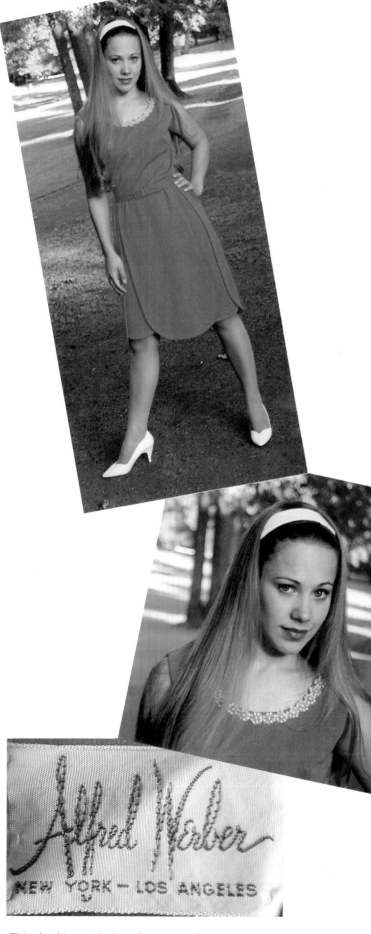

This shocking pink dress features a "flower-petal" overskirt and a typically-sixties bead-trimmed neckline. *Courtesy of Persona Vintage Clothing.*

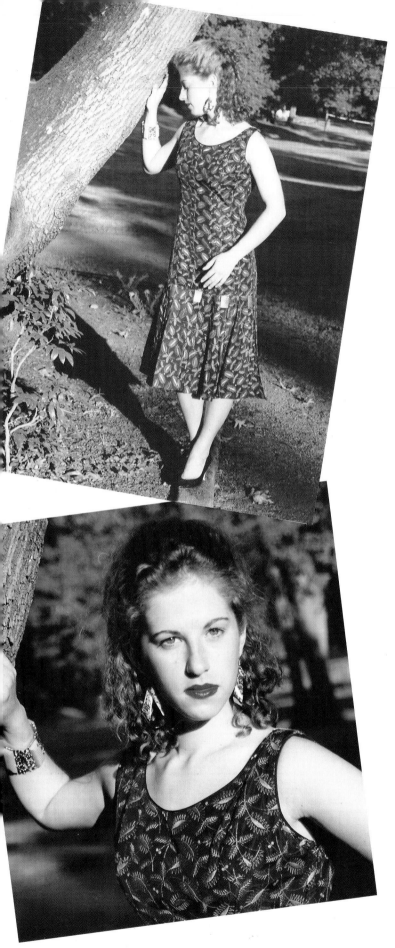

As years passed, the mini got "minier," sometimes barely covering young women "decently." Nonetheless, the mini lost its shocking effect on the older generation soon enough, and designer Mary Quant was allowed into Buckingham Palace wearing a mini in 1966. When the mini was no longer considered suitably shocking enough to the older generation, the maxi gained favor—and became an eyebrow-raiser simply because it was the longest skirt seen since the teens. Even *Life* magazine noted the transition with a huge cover photograph and the headline: "The Mini or the Maxi?" First worn in 1969, the maxi owed its success in large part to the trendy women who had been donning "granny" styles since mid-decade. Made up of shawls, high-top laced boots, long and full skirts, and faux petticoats, the granny look started out as a fad worn by a small group of women. Much to the surprise of most designers, however, the style caught on, and by the late sixties couture designers were copying the street-found style which would become the hallmark of the 1970s. Perhaps, like the childish baby doll dress, the granny look acted as a form of reassurance to men during a time of strident feminism. (Women, after all, didn't wish to be viewed as Amazons—so see how cute I look in this baby doll dress? See how feminine and old-fashioned I look in this granny dress? Reassuring men has been the aim of more than one fashion trend. "It is the custom that whenever a woman has made some notable advance into man's domain she will reassure him by adopting, for a spell, an ultra-feminine style of dress," C. Willett Cunnington, one of the early historical fashion experts, noted in his *Englishwomen's Clothing in the 19th Century*.)

Too, the granny look was the first true fashion that came from the streets, not couture designers—a trend that had a profound effect in the sixties and seventies, when the Beatnik, hippie, and flower-child looks would rise to fame—also from the streets.

Relaxing Standards

Increasingly, casual wear was becoming the thing to wear most of the time; not that standards had become as relaxed as those found today—but where once a woman wouldn't think of attending school, going into town, or doing other everyday activities such as going to the hairdresser or grocery store in anything but a nice dress or skirt and blouse, the woman of the sixties increasingly found herself feeling perfectly acceptable doing such activities dressed in slacks. Even Emily Post, always on the conservative side of

A stunning taffeta dress with all-over turquoise embroidery and wide satin insertion ribbon. *Courtesy of Persona Vintage Clothing.*

things, agreed that women with figures suited to slacks were perfectly within good taste. "Slacks as sports wear have been accepted for a number of years," she noted in 1969. "They are certainly the most practical dress for an active woman engaging in sailing, hunting, heavy housework, gardening, or many other activities." But, the queen of manners cautioned, "unless the wearer is reasonably slim they are anything but flattering. The same is true of evening slacks and the popular 'pants suits.' They cannot be surpassed for comfort, and for smartness worn by the right woman, but on anyone else a long 'at home' skirt, or a cocktail or dinner dress is far more appealing."

In keeping with this new relaxed atmosphere, for the first time elasticized fashions meant for more than just sportswear emerged, as did traditional Levi's made specifically for women. "Hipsters," pants (or even skirts)

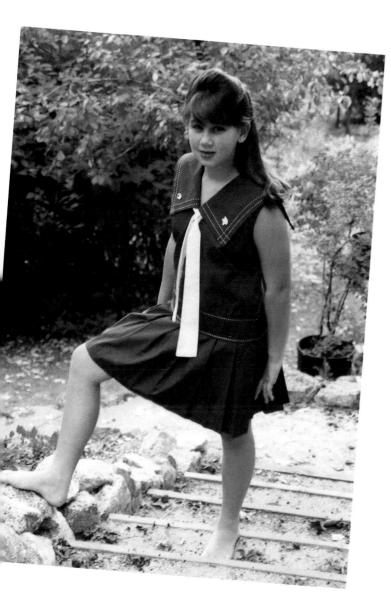

A 1920s-revival dress in the classic sailor style. *Courtesy of The Very Little Theatre.*

cut to end just below the waistline, and fitted around the hips, also appeared in the late 1960s, as did trouser outfits or pants suits. The latter were the first real attempt since the 1920s (when little success was achieved) to make trousers for women something to be worn in place of a day dress. Considerably more dressy than any pair of jeans, and even the more classy Capris, pantsuits usually featured a matching blouse and jacket or vest. Still, they were not greeted with a communal cheer. "I remember in 1968 I came up with a collection of tunic dresses over pants," sportswear designer Stan Herman recalls. "Mildred Custin [then president of Bonwit Teller's]...sat in her big office and said 'No way. It's not going to work. They'll never let women into restaurants wearing these.'" She was right, many restaurants did refuse women in such outfits, but women didn't seem to mind, and were soon wearing them elsewhere.

In 1964 the topless bathing suit was introduced. As would be expected, it created a media uproar—but was never adopted by more than a few élan women. In the world of mainstream swimwear, the bikini (considerably scantier than its 1950s predecessor) could be seen on nearly any beach. Any uplifts, girdles, or waist-nippers found in the fifties disappeared by the mid-sixties—the new look being *eau natural*—even at the expense of the poor soul who managed to squeeze herself into the suit. As *Vogue* put it in 1968: "The minimum two piece for a perfect tan, leaving the least possible marks from sunbathing," was what was now desired. Nonetheless, in 1967, probably in reaction to what she saw on the streets, Emily Post insisted: "Never wear shorts or a bathing suit on the street...in most communities it is actually illegal to appear dressed in this way."

The formerly-worshipped Lastex (first appearing in bathing suits in the 1920s) was rarely used anymore, the new Spandex and Lycra being considerably stronger. "When its dried in the sun it's a sinuous velvety black, and when it's soaked with water it glistens like a seal on the rocks," *Vogue* rhapsodized about the latter.

Like most other things in the sixties, accessories remained largely the same as they had in the fifties—with only a few slight changes. Stiletto (or "spike") heels were still favorites—though (undoubtedly having seen far too many women teetering on them) Emily Post noted in 1965 that even if a lady is short "it is better to wear a moderate heel than a 'spike' if one is unable to walk gracefully on the latter." Gloves were also still worn, and Ms. Post had plenty to say about that, too:

"*Gloves are worn on city streets, to luncheons, dinner parties, and other social gatherings, to*

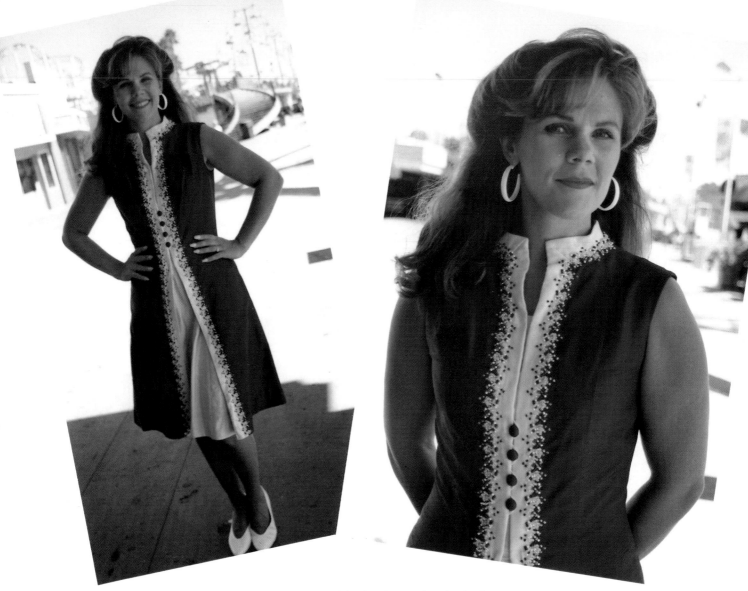

With style lines inspired by the Orient, this Elizabeth Byrne 100% silk dress features two rows of beading running from the shoulder to the hem. The label indicates it was "tailored in Hong Kong." *Courtesy of The Very Little Theatre.*

churches, restaurants, theaters, and all other public places of entertainment. At a restaurant, theater, or the like, they may be removed on arrival, but they are generally left on in church except during communion or when it is very warm...Gloves which come above the elbow are worn only with sleeveless or strapless evening dresses. Wrist-length or three-quarter length gloves are correct with less formal gowns. At informal dances it is not necessary to wear gloves at all if you prefer not to do so."

But unlike the gloves worn in the 1950s, which could be both elegant and whimsical, most women chose plain little white gloves—à la Jackie Kennedy. (Some women even dispensed with gloves altogether; Kezia Keeble notes that when she was a new and young editor at *Glamour* in 1964, her editor-in-chief Kathleen Casey was shocked after reviewing some

recent photos Keeble had helped shoot for the magazine. "Where are the white gloves?" Casey asked. When Keeble replied that many young women, herself included, never wore them anymore, Casey retorted: "Then you are not a lady.")

In 1961, the First Lady also inspired another fashion: pillbox hats. Though pillboxes had been worn in the 1950s and before, unlike the fifties version (which were curved to fit the head, rather like an upside-down bowl), the new versions were true pillboxes—perfectly round and perched atop the head. In keeping with Mrs. Kennedy's penchant for simple clothing, pillboxes were very simple and rarely had anything more than a slight veil as trimming. Still, hats were not the obligatory things they once were. "If you look well in hats, wear them. A well-chosen hat may add dash and distinction to your outfit that a bare head can't possibly achieve," Emily Post advised.

"If you are one of the many women who feel that there is no hat in the world becoming to you, settle for a little veil or a band or bow on those occasions when it is necessary to cover your head. You must wear a hat to all Roman Catholic ceremonies, and it is always correct at churches of every faith. At official luncheons and receptions they are almost a requirement, and beyond that, hats may be, and are, worn at any time and on any occasion that you wish during the day. A small hat or veil is appropriate, but not necessary, with a cocktail dress. Except for the necessary head covering at an evening wedding, a hat, even the smallest veil, is never worn with an evening dress."

At any rate, hats were growing ever more difficult to perch atop increasingly towering beehive hairdos.

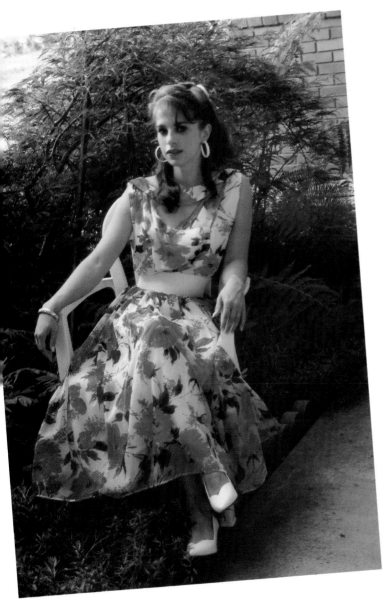

A softly draped chiffon dress with bold poppies blazing across it. *Courtesy of The Very Little Theatre.*

Paper Penchant

"After all, who is going to do laundry in space?" one textile designer summed up the most novel trend of the sixties. In an era where the old-fashioned view of having lasting, classic clothes was dying out, and the modern idea of carefree, easy clothes was rushing in, paper clothes seemed just the thing. Actually, like the granny style, paper clothes were a surprise to almost everybody—certainly to couture designers. The first smashing success paper dress was actually sold in 1966 by Scott Paper Company. By sending in $1, women could receive Scott's "Paper Caper" dress, plus 52¢ worth of coupons for Scott paper towels, cups, tissues, etcetera. A simple, chemise-style dress in a red paisley design or black and white "op art" pattern, to the company's amazement, they sold 500,000! Around the same time, Hallmark began selling "hostess dresses" of paper which were created to match paper party napkins and tablecloths. Paper maternity wear suddenly popped up, as did paper wedding dresses (you only wear it once, anyway, right?).

Soon, ads advised women that for two wrappers from Dove, Lux, or Lifeboy soap, plus $1, anyone could own a "Swinging Dress" and hat of paper. Breck offered a dress for $1.25 plus a box top from Go Go Light high lighter. Even Pillsbury offered a dress for $1 and a box top. In 1967, the paper dress seemed so practical and modern, it was predicted that by 1980, 25% of all money spent on clothing would go toward the purchase of paper clothes. The convenience seemed too good to be true. If a dress was too long, just whip out your scissors and cut it shorter; if it stained, throw it out; if you tired of it, dump it in the trash! Paper dresses from clothing stores easily cost under $15 (although one designer, Judith Brewer, is reported to have created a coat made up of paper pom-poms, costing some $200), and home-sewers could buy kits for paper dresses that only required a few seams be stitched up; some companies even offered dresses that could be decorated by their buyer with pens, paints, rhinestones, and other trimmings.

"The Big Paper Craze" was one of *Mademoiselle's* cover stories in June of 1967. "In terms of how much pow you get for your pennies, the paper dress is the ultimate smart-money fashion," the editors praised. "And the news in the paper is this: surprisingly pretty prints, clever new shapes that would do credit to an origami expert. (Surprisingly long life, too: as many as 12 outings.)" Actually paper dresses were a little more than just paper; usually composed of 93% cel-

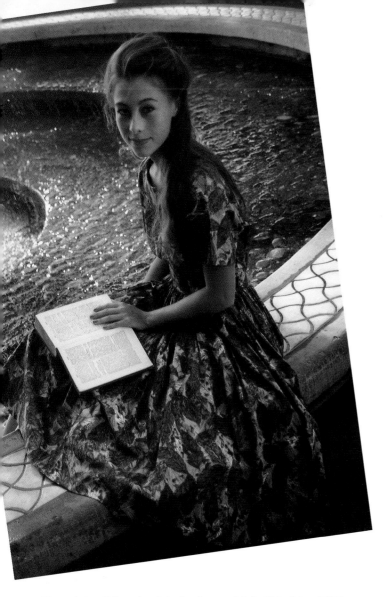

Though it still has the tight bodice and full skirt of the 1950s, this dress can be dated to the sixties by its unfussed design and color scheme. Its skirt is also supported by an attached Pellon slip (as opposed to having Pellon sticking to the entire back of the fashion fabric), which is more typical of the 1960s, when skirt width began to decline and full crinolines went out of favor for daywear.

lulose and 7% nylon (rather like dry baby wipes), or sometimes made up of "Dura-Weve®", which was another blend of cellulose reinforced with rayon, they were not likely to rip at the slightest move. Many paper clothes also featured closures of Velcro®, making them seem even more "space-age." Ads for paper clothes varied considerably in this paper-crazed issue of *Mademoiselle*: Tuscancy offered a dress for $7, Tiger Tissue offered a dress designed by Felix Safian for $6, Mars of Asheville, a dress for $1.75, Scott, a dress for $6, James Sterling Paper Fashion, a dress for $9.

Mademoiselle's copy—headlined "Paper Profits"—highlighted a variety of paper fashions, made from intriguing and creative materials. "Smart Smock," one

garment was dubbed. "What's surprising? Item: this smock's a tube of paper. *Paper*. Not only that, but—item: it is paper that's been knitted. *Knitted*. That means a new kind of texture. And not only is it surprising, but item: it's spiffy-looking....$8" Another section noted other surprises: "The floppy paper hat (surprise! paper hats aren't just for parties), $4...Who says a paper dress has to be shaped like a paper bag? Right now, designers are getting all kinds of new ideas down on paper—everything from bikinis to bedroom slippers..." to pillowcases for $1.35, to aprons and laundry bags for $1.75, to "two scraps of brown/white Kaycel [a papery-like rayon], elasticized around for a teeny-weeny sun bikini...$5," to clog shoes for $15, earrings for $12, scuff slippers ("when they've had it, kick them off—and out") for 60¢, and "possibly the flightiest shoes around; metallic Kaycel—gold scrolled with pink—threaded with shiny pink ribbon...$6." Another innovative dress was advertised as: "Party Stopper. Shimmering white mini with silver fringe. Polyplastic on Scott Dura-Weve® paper. Wipe off and press again and again. $5.95 ppd." But without a doubt, the weirdest paper dress—by one of the wackiest dress manufacturers of the sixties—was meant to grow herbs. "It was amazing," Paraphernalia's founder admits. "There were little seeds planted in a kind of blotter paper, very soft—kind of like a Handi-Wipe. It was like those Magic Rocks you put in water. When you watered the dress, it grew these strange little blossoms."

So hot were paper fashions that Mars Manufacturing reverted from producing stockings to creating paper clothes; Abraham & Straus opened paper clothes boutiques; Saks Fifth Avenue opened a paper fashion department, as did Lord & Taylor, Altman's, Bonwit Teller, Gimble's...Within a few years, however, the paper fashion industry was in real danger of extinction. It's final cause of death? Not, as we might imagine today, because disposable clothing was wasteful—but because the clothing was so easily apt to catch fire. Even if *Mademoiselle* had featured a solution to that problem: "So what's new? A crisp, little paper tent...fire-resistant paper." And for a mere $3.

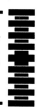

"The look a man likes...curves and planes perfectly placed for glamour by the famous Jantzen figure experts who know what it takes to make a girl gorgeous." - Jantzen ad, May 1957.

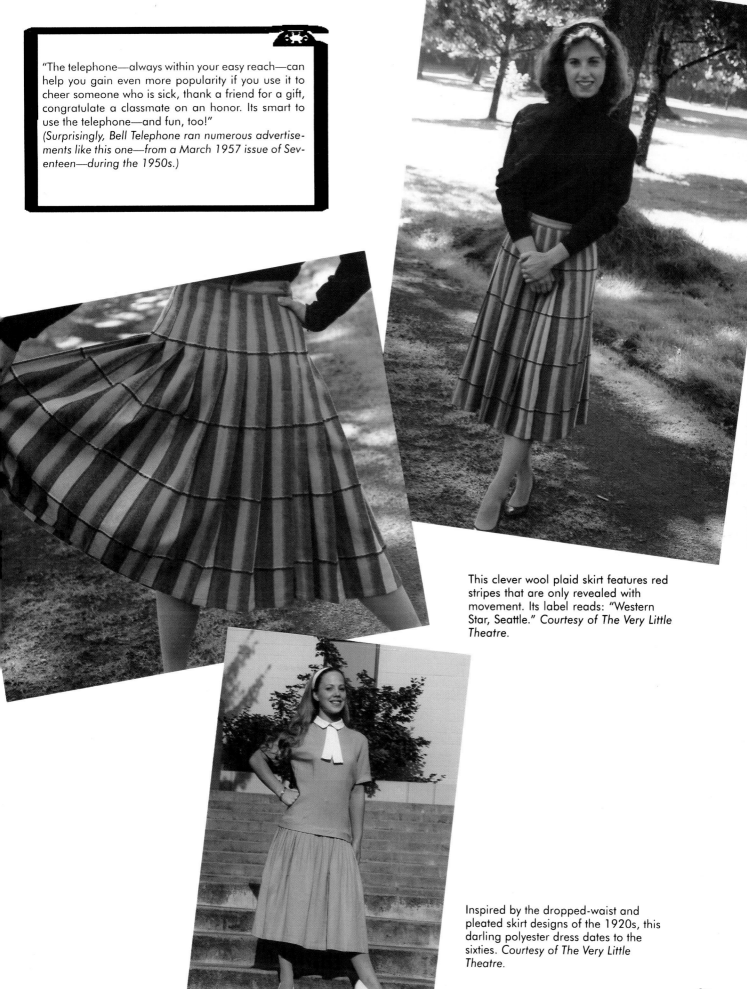

"The telephone—always within your easy reach—can help you gain even more popularity if you use it to cheer someone who is sick, thank a friend for a gift, congratulate a classmate on an honor. Its smart to use the telephone—and fun, too!"
(Surprisingly, Bell Telephone ran numerous advertisements like this one—from a March 1957 issue of Seventeen—during the 1950s.)

This clever wool plaid skirt features red stripes that are only revealed with movement. Its label reads: "Western Star, Seattle." *Courtesy of The Very Little Theatre.*

Inspired by the dropped-waist and pleated skirt designs of the 1920s, this darling polyester dress dates to the sixties. *Courtesy of The Very Little Theatre.*

95

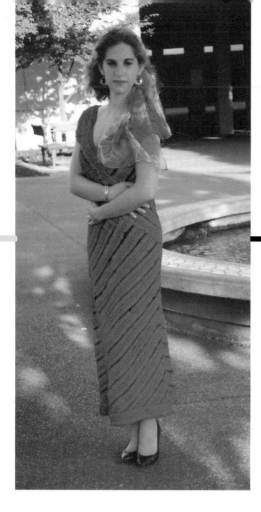

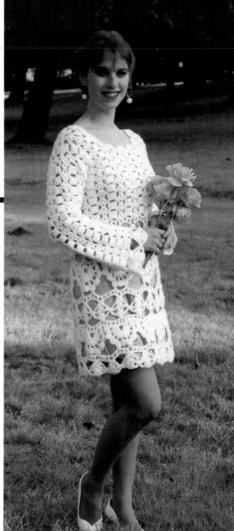

A crocheted dress from the late sixties. The original owner remembers having a variety of different colored slips to wear beneath it. *Courtesy of Jerri Bickmore.*

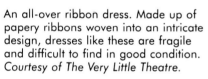

An all-over ribbon dress. Made up of papery ribbons woven into an intricate design, dresses like these are fragile and difficult to find in good condition. *Courtesy of The Very Little Theatre.*

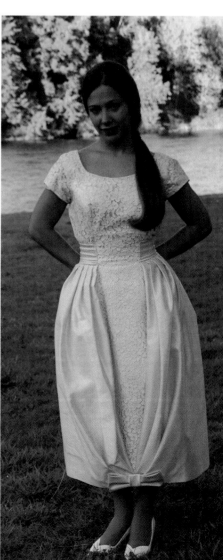

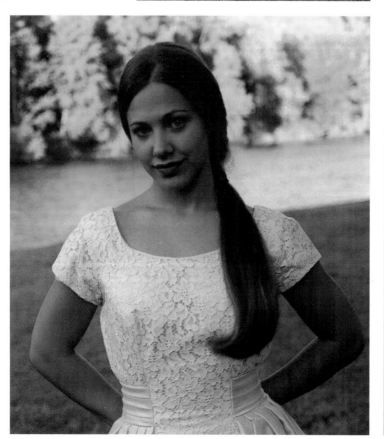

Of ecru satin woven with gold, this Chinese-inspired dress came with a matching jacket. *Courtesy of The Very Little Theatre.*

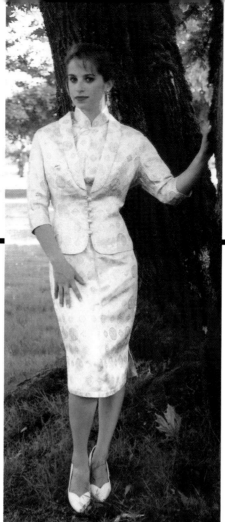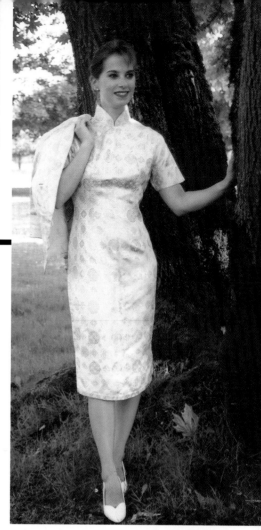

A "bubble" dress of silk and lace with a Jane Cindre label. *Courtesy of Persona Vintage Clothing.*

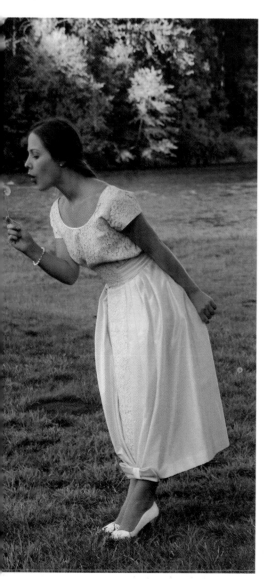

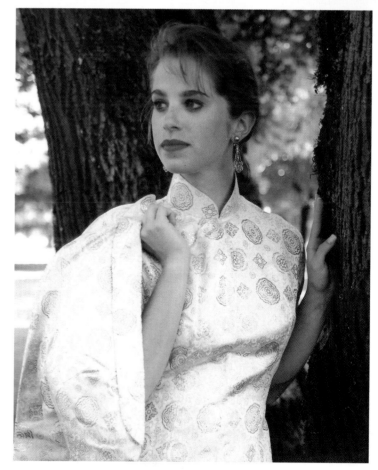

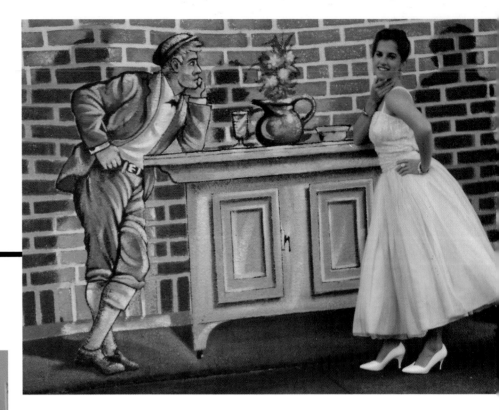

Though most garments made in the Orient featured extensive beading and other hand-applied trims, this relatively simple chiffon and lace evening gown features a Hong Kong label. *Courtesy of The Very Little Theatre.*

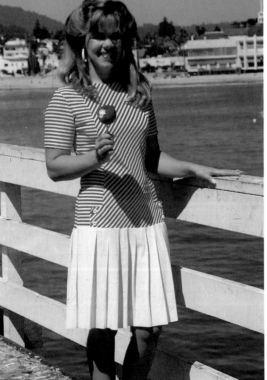

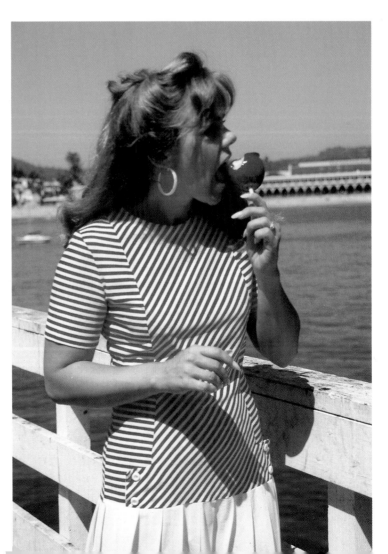

This polyester dropped waist dress with its plain, short, pleated skirt makes clever use of stripes. *Courtesy of The Very Little Theatre.*

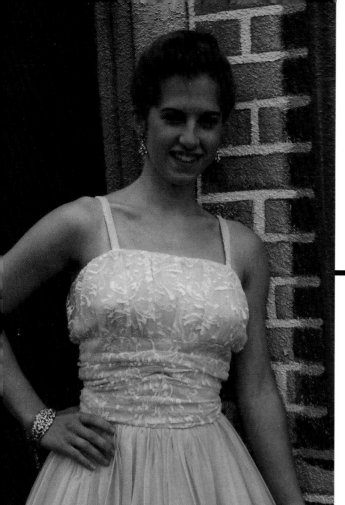

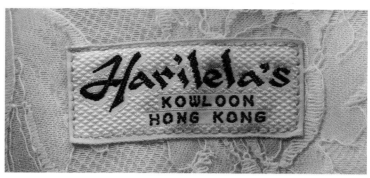

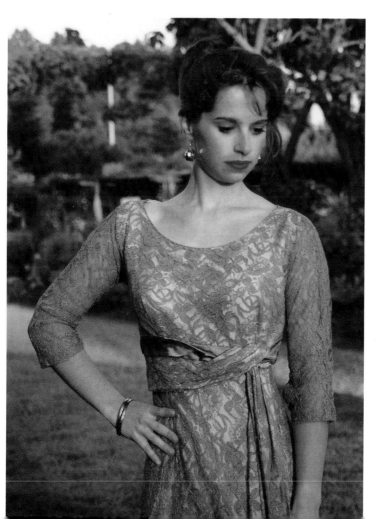

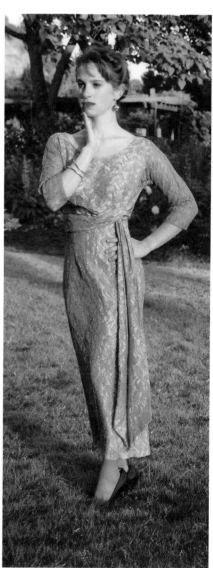

A simple but stunning evening dress from the 1960s, made up of milk-chocolate all-over lace with satin accents.

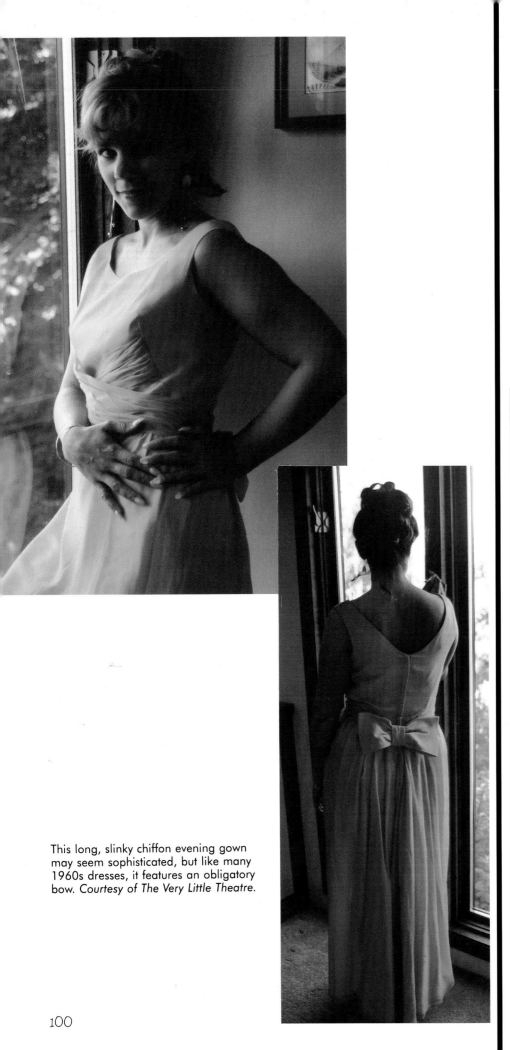

An evening gown inspired by the sleek, simple lines popularized by Jackie Kennedy. This dress is actually two piece: A simple, plain gown with wide straps and a plain neckline, and a beaded over-top fastening in the back with hooks and eyes. *Courtesy of Marianine's Vintage Chic.*

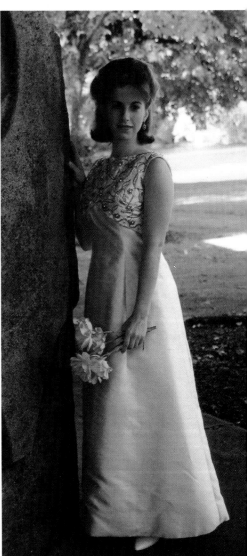

This long, slinky chiffon evening gown may seem sophisticated, but like many 1960s dresses, it features an obligatory bow. *Courtesy of The Very Little Theatre.*

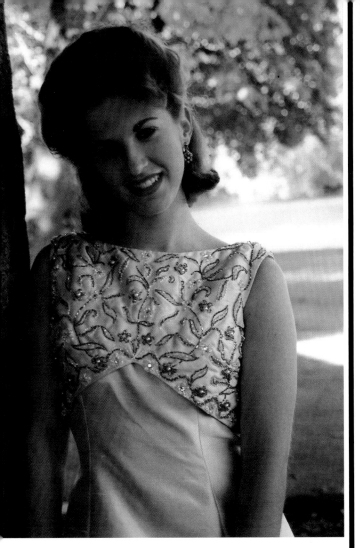

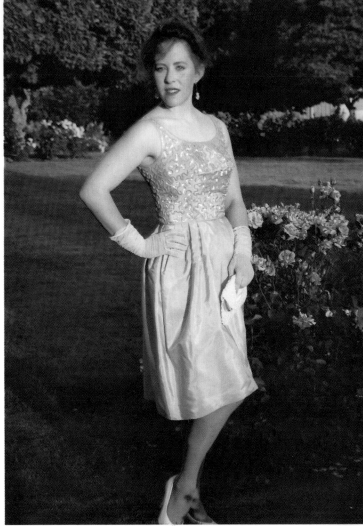

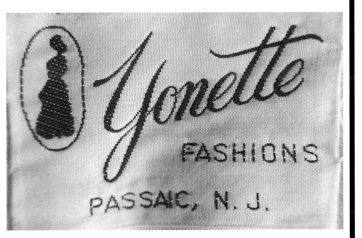

Yonette
FASHIONS
PASSAIC, N. J.

"[The average woman's] fashion needs are similar to those of most working girls. She likes good separates and casual dresses...something less casual for movies, dinner or theatre dates. Her call for very formal clothes is small (she didn't wear one full-length gown last year), but she does like to get dressed up for informal dances and parties...she keeps a shoe wardrobe of three basic pumps—black, tan and navy..."
- *Ladies Home Journal*, 1959.

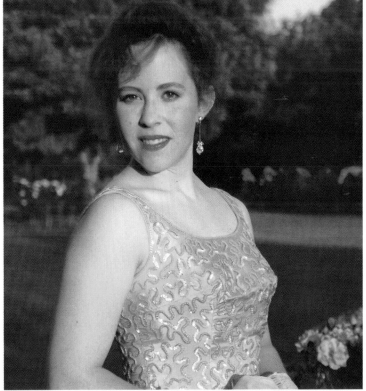

This pink taffeta evening dress features a sequined bodice and a Jr. Theme label. *Courtesy of The Very Little Theatre.*

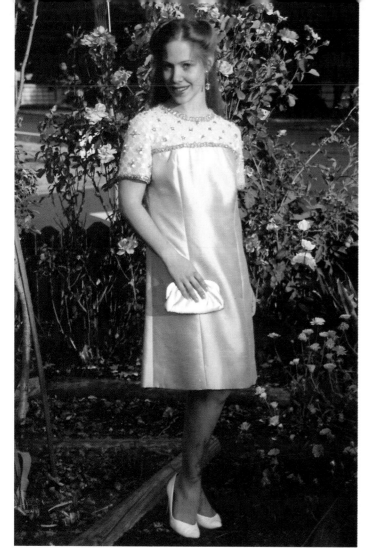

A party or cocktail ensemble consisting of a raw silk, sparkling silver dress with a yolk of netting, braid trim, and beading, plus a matching raw silk jacket. Designed by a relatively unknown designer ("Mr. Frank," sold by The Addis Co.), it is nonetheless a stunning example of ready-to-wear at its best. With bound buttonholes, covered snaps, and fine finishing details, this dress rivals couture ready-to-wear. *Courtesy of Persona Vintage Clothing.*

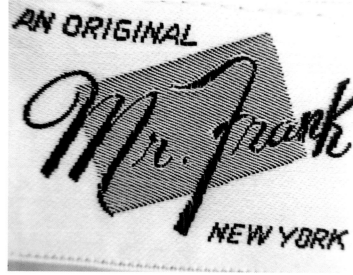

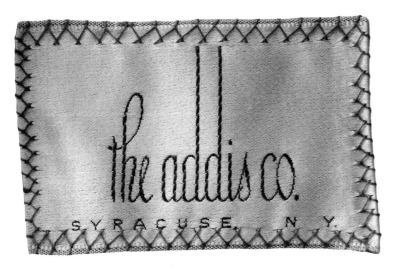

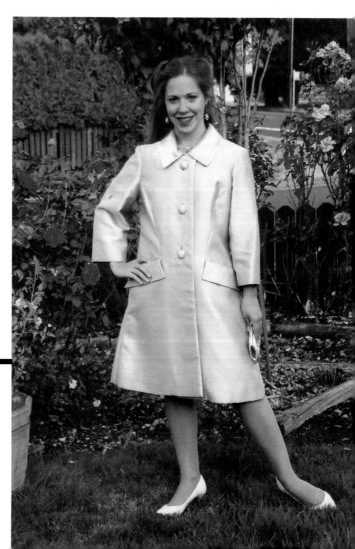

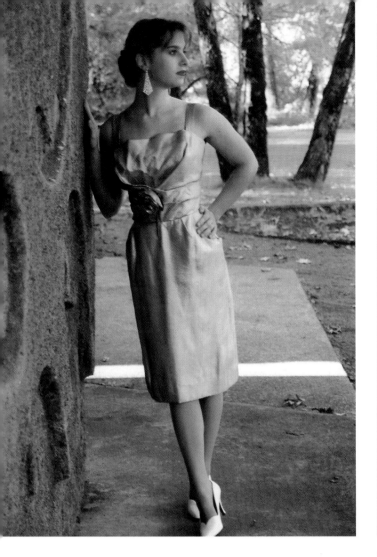

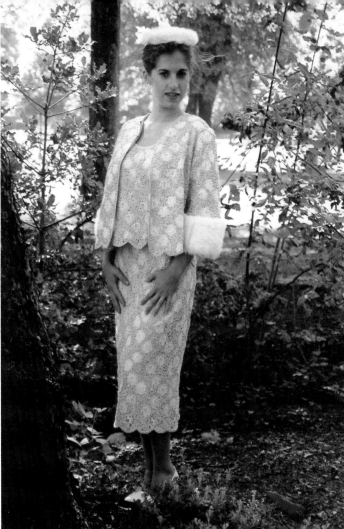

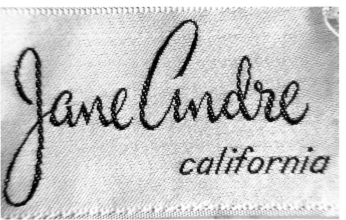

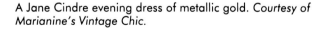

A Jane Cindre evening dress of metallic gold. *Courtesy of Marianine's Vintage Chic.*

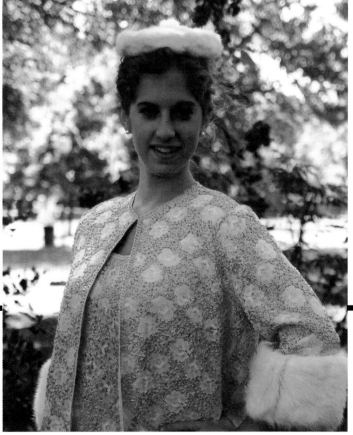

Made up of finely ruched ribbon, lace, and fur, this skirt with a matching blouse and jacket was a bride's going-away outfit. The original owner, Mary Mason, remembers she purchased the ensemble near the end of July in 1966 at The Desert Inn Hotel dress shop in Las Vegas, Nevada, for about $150. "I told the clerk I wanted something beautiful, something spiffy," Mary recalls. "She said, 'One moment—' and brought this out of the back room."

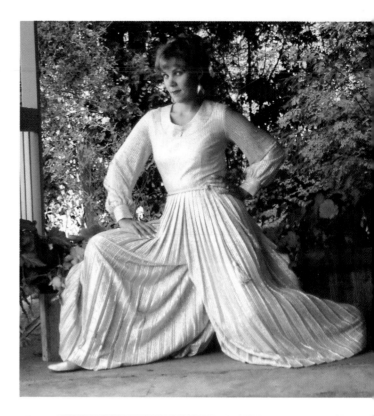

> "Fashion is not a funny hat. Fashion is a business that affects not only the way we look but the way we live and think. New York is undeniably the fashion center of the United States. The whole ready-to-wear industry (which is young—about 35 years old), is located in a concentrated area, six blocks long and three blocks wide. Responsible for more than a billion-and-a-half dollars' worth of business, it gives employment to 179,545 women and a like number of men. It is the fashion trades that have given women who work an opportunity to create jobs where their special skills and aptitudes can be used and developed without stint."
> - Charm, "Fashion is Their Business," June 1955.

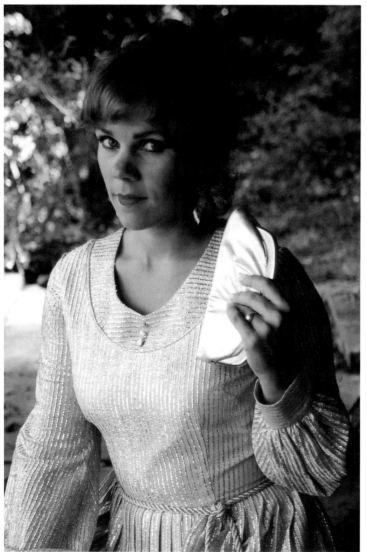

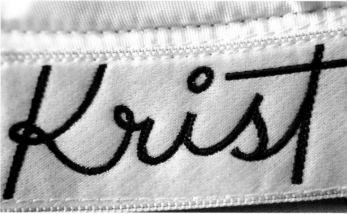

A late 1960s evening outfit by Krist. This is actually a pantsuit, but was considered acceptable for expensive restaurants because its extremely wide legs made it appear to be a dress except upon close examination. Of metallic fabric with tiny raised stripes, the outfit is finished off with its original silver-metallic rope belt, slipper-like silver metallic shoes, and clutch.

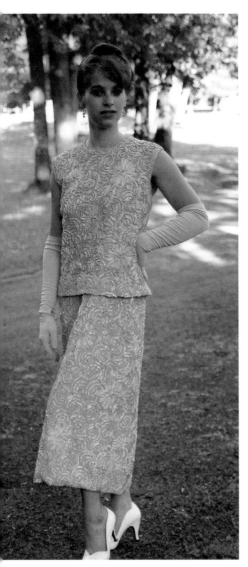

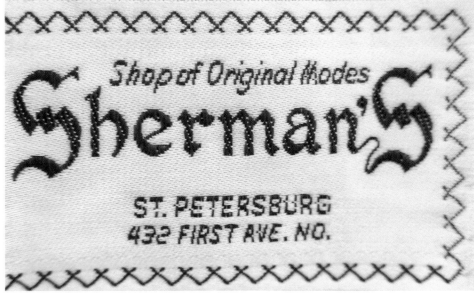

Shop of Original Modes

Sherman'S

ST. PETERSBURG
432 FIRST AVE. NO.

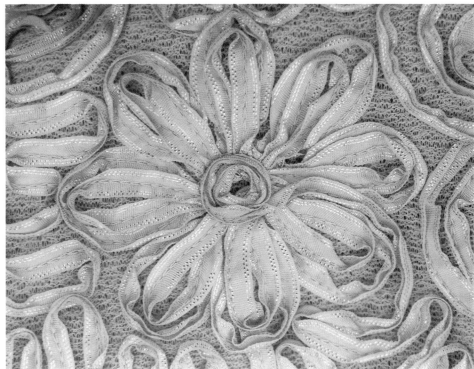

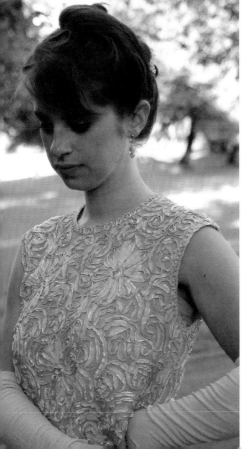

From the 1960s, this magnificent two-piece Sherman evening dress features all-over braid work in an intricate design. *Courtesy of The Very Little Theatre.*

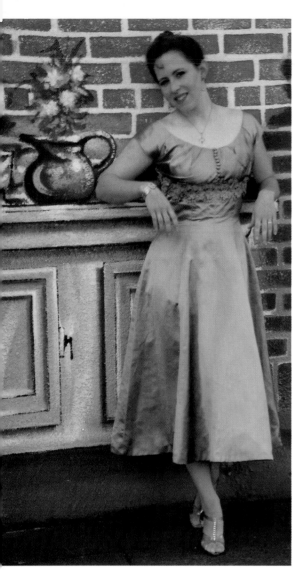

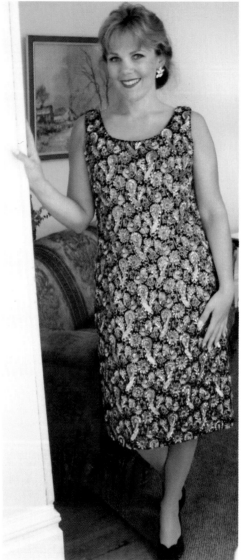

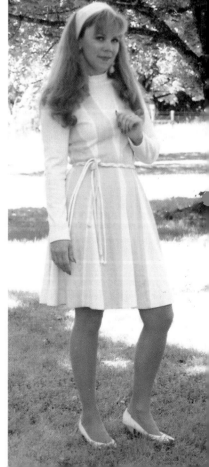

Though evening dresses remained much the same in the 1960s as they had in the 1950s, they were generally less fussy. This lovely dress is by Emma Dombe. *Courtesy of The Very Little Theatre.*

A stunning chemise dress from the 1960s with an all-over beaded design. *Courtesy of The Very Little Theatre.*

A 1960s knit day dress with pieced yellow and white stripes and a matching woven rope belt.

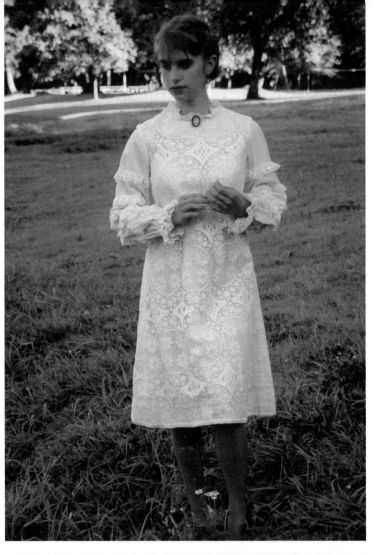

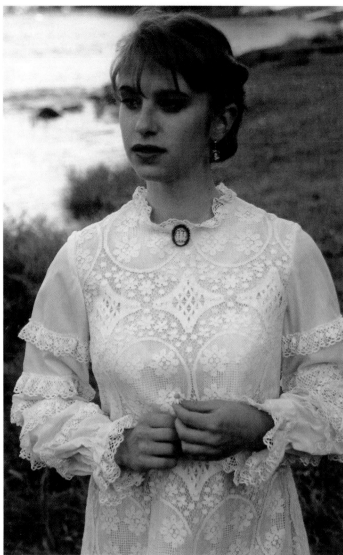

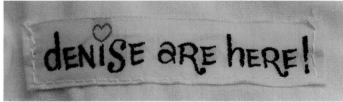

Though this dress (with a "Denise are here!" label) has a 1970s feel to it, it is actually a forerunner to the longer-skirted "granny" dresses of that decade and dates to c. 1968-69. The dress also features a relatively modern invention: The plastic zipper, just coming into regular use by the end of the sixties. *Courtesy of Jerri Bickmore.*

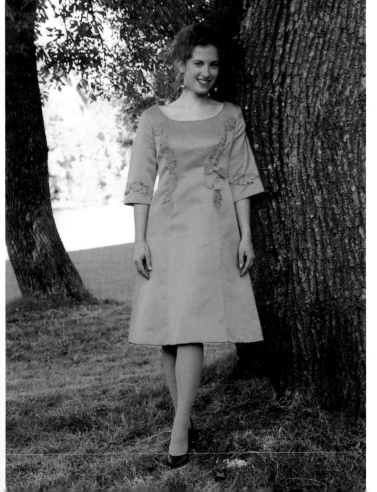

A trapeze dress of silk. *Courtesy of Persona Vintage Clothing.*

A Joan Miller dress of wool with attached black knit collar and cuffs. *Courtesy of Persona Vintage Clothing.*

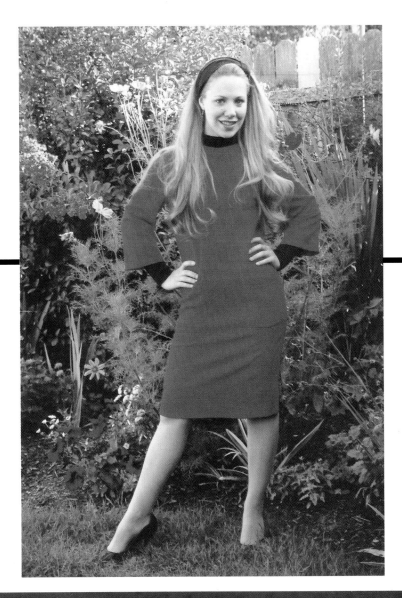

A late sixties dress, hinting at the ruffled "granny" styles that would sweep through the 1970s. Of peachy taffeta covered with all-over lace, this dress features a sewn-on cameo at the neckline. *Courtesy of Diane Seldman.*

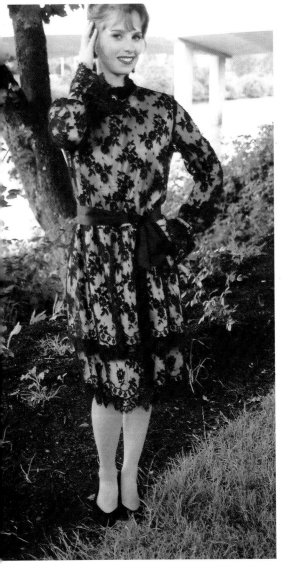

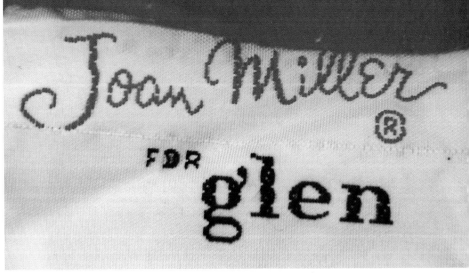

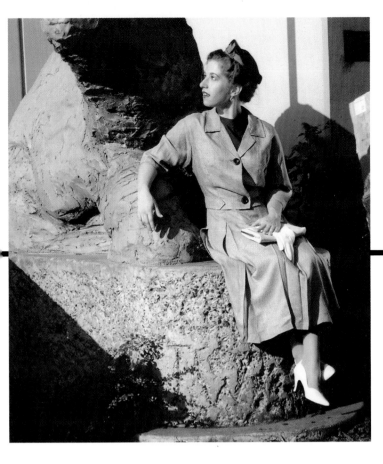

A suit-like dress featuring a pleated skirt with an attached, solid-colored, sleeveless bodice, and a separate, matching jacket. *Courtesy of The Very Little Theatre.*

A classy knit outfit, consisting of a sweater and pleated skirt. The label reads: "Castleberry, London, New York." *Courtesy of The Very Little Theatre.*

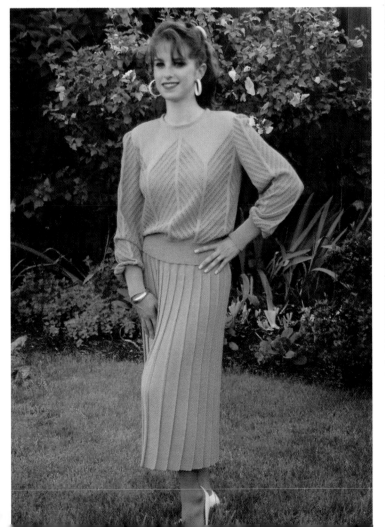

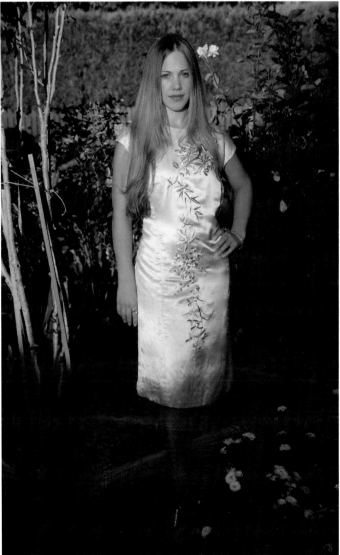

An exceptional chemise dress from the 1960s. Made of silk satin, it carries no label, and has many couture designer details (including a hand applied lining); however, it is most likely this dress was home-made (or made by a local dress-maker) of great skill. *Courtesy of The Very Little Theatre.*

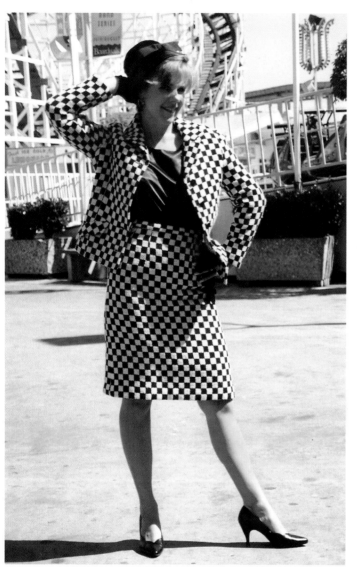

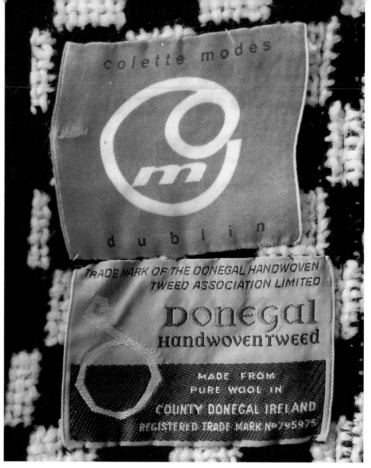

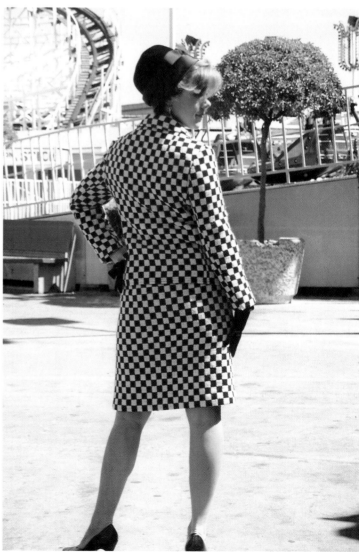

A Chanel-inspired knit suit of playful checks, made in Dublin. *Courtesy of The Very Little Theatre.*

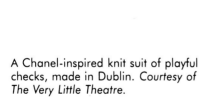

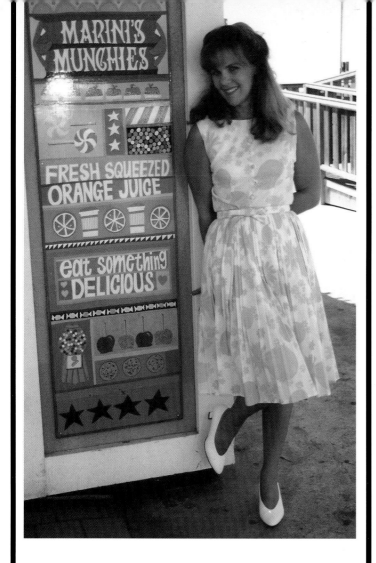

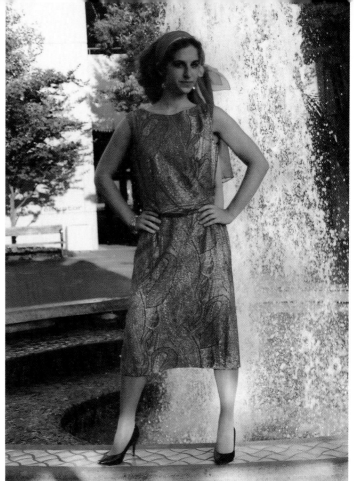

In the 1960s, this sort of playful polyester print "everyday" dress was exceedingly common, but today such dresses are difficult to come by in good condition. This dress features a "Stacy Ames of the four sisters" label. *Courtesy of The Very Little Theatre.*

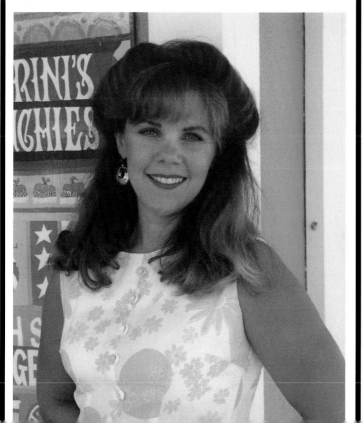

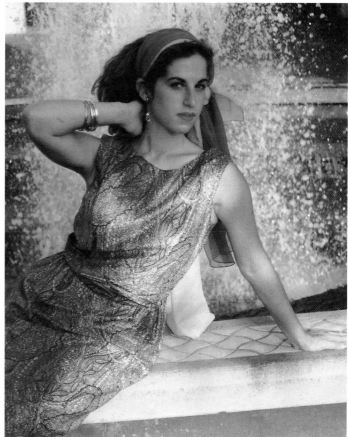

An exceptional metallic party dress dating to the 1960s but finding inspiration in the flapper styles of the 1920s. *Courtesy of The Very Little Theatre.*

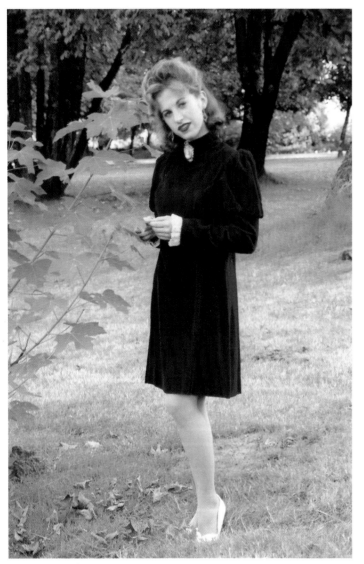

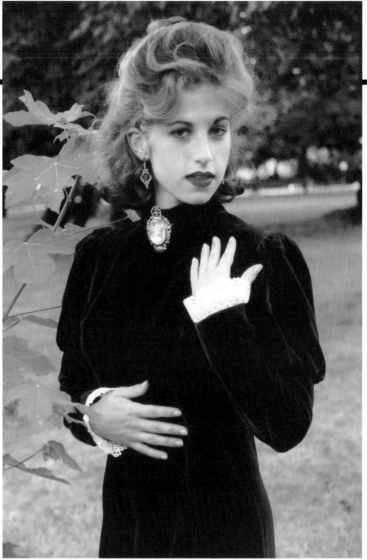

A c.1968-69 "Young Edwardian" velvet party dress trimmed with crochet lace. *Courtesy of Jerri Bickmore.*

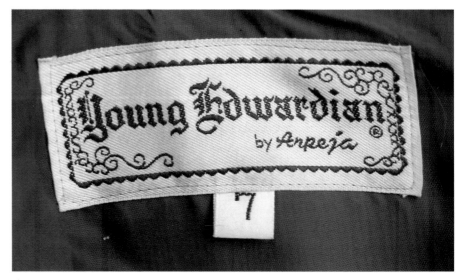

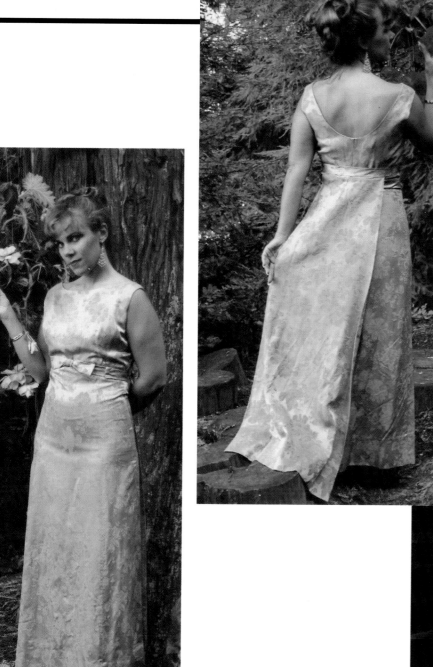

A simple but lovely brocade evening gown featuring a decorative back flap, giving the air of a train without the hassle. *Courtesy of* The Very Little Theatre.

A two-piece evening dress featuring a simple chemise dress of taffeta overlaid with all-over matching lace. The overskirt is separate and attached to the belt. Originally, this overskirt may have been a bubble skirt (or it may have been updated and altered to be a bubble skirt, then restored to its original shape). *Courtesy of* The Very Little Theatre.

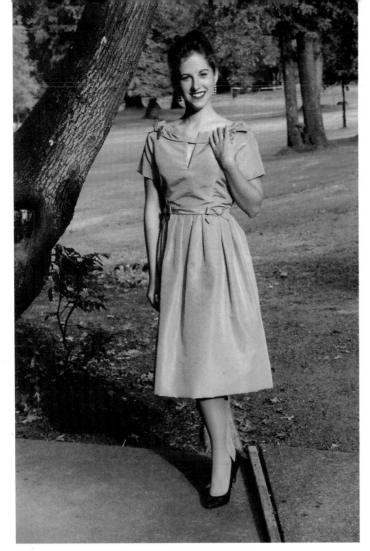

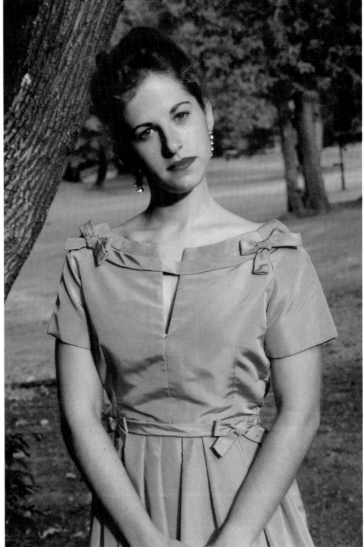

A Christian Dior dress (#32219) of heavy, corded taffeta. The inside reveals typically Dior features: A complete, attached slip closing with its own hooks and eyes, an inner waistband belt, and another row of hooks and eyes closing the dress. The dress features both Dior's label and a Harrod's (London) department store label. This dress dates to after Dior's death; custom designs actually created by Dior himself sell for thousands at affluent auction houses. *Courtesy of Flossy McGrew's.*

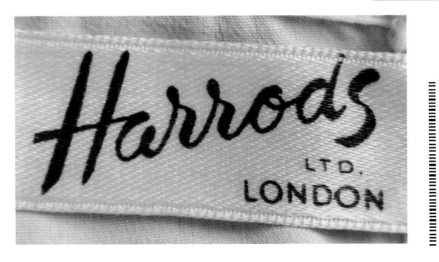

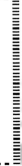

"Now! Say good-bye to uncomfortable garters! Introducing Ultra Hold, the most exciting fashion news of the day! UltraHold is the new liquid roll on applicator that is applied to your legs to hold up your stockings all day long without garters! Your stockings stay up comfortably...without garters! No most costly snags or tears...no more uncomfortable pulling or pinching...it's the most important breakthrough in convenience and savings in years!...only $4."
- UltraHold ad, 1967.

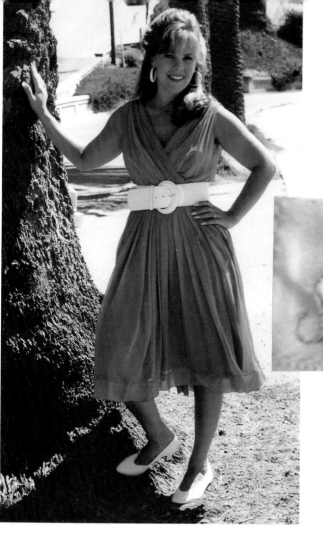

A draped chiffon evening dress with a Sax Fifth Avenue label. *Courtesy of The Very Little Theatre.*

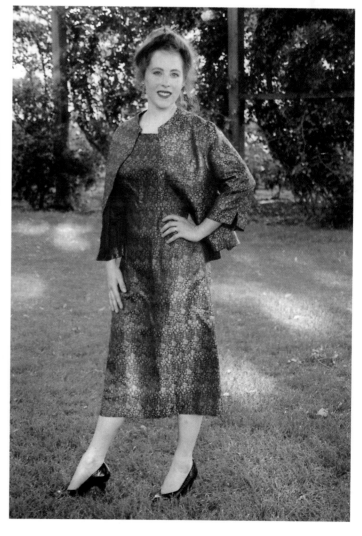

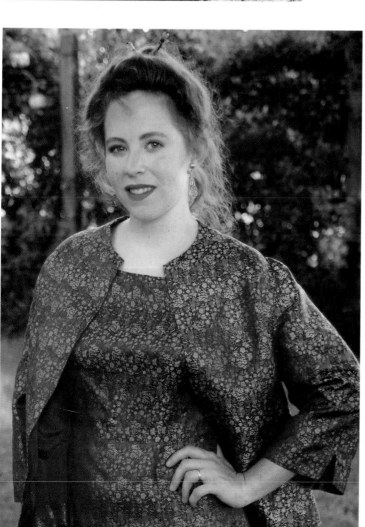

A very fine quality, woven print, Chinese-style dress with a matching jacket. *Courtesy of The Very Little Theatre.*

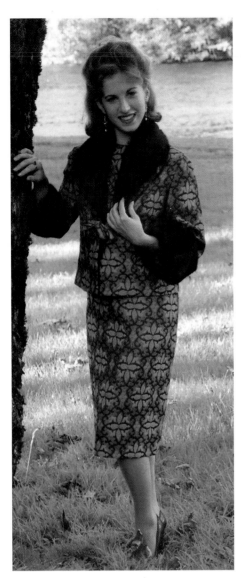

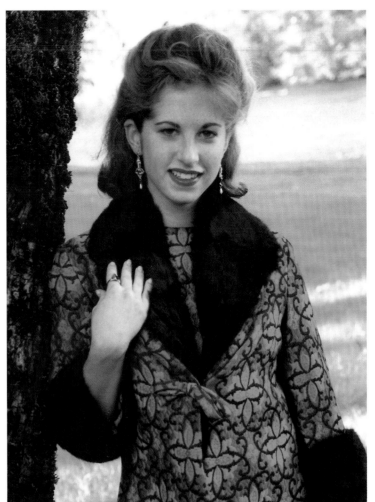

A magnificent suit of green brocade, trimmed with mink. *Courtesy of Marianine's Vintage Chic.*

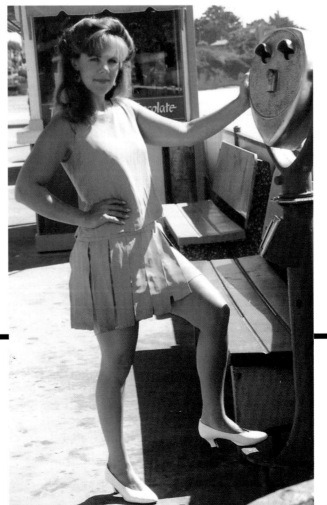

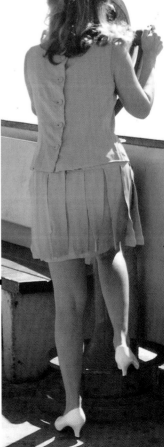

This two-piece dress of rayon was inspired by fringed 1920s flapper styles, and contains a "Saba Jrs." label. *Courtesy of The Very Little Theatre.*

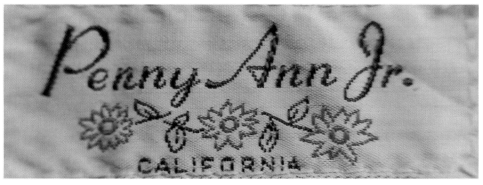

A wonderfully sixties Peggy Ann Jr. dress with a plastic zipper running down the back—something rarely seen in 1950s and early 1960s dresses. *Courtesy of Jerri Bickmore.*

"What to wear with your new wig: chiffon culottes."
- *Vogue, 1962.*

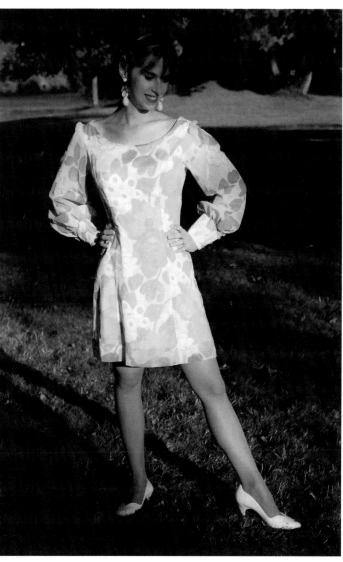

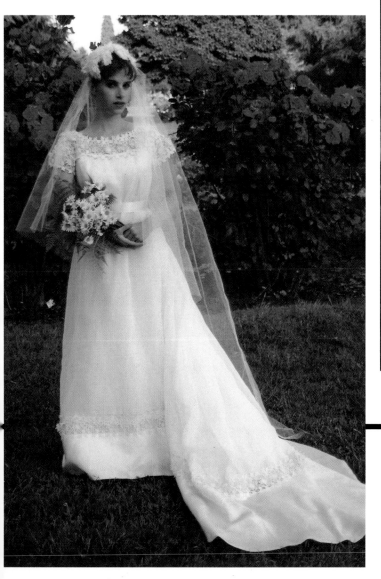

A 1960s bridal gown of taffeta and chiffon, featuring lace in a daisy pattern.

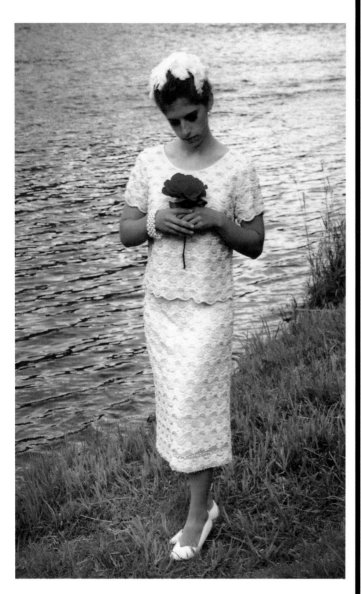

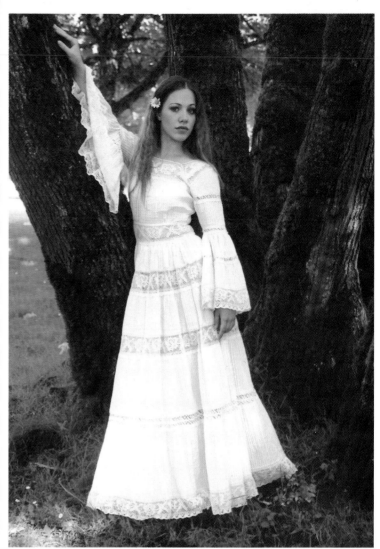

This elegant 1960s two-piece bridal dress is entirely beaded. *Courtesy of The Very Little Theatre.*

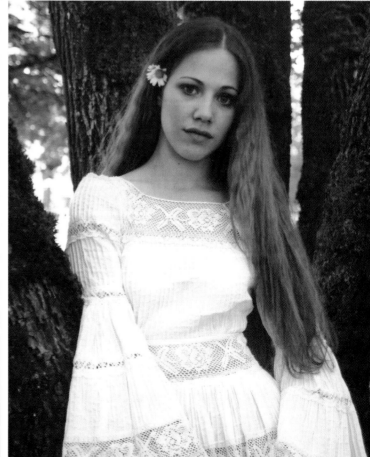

Dating to c. 1969-70, this home-made dress (probably a wedding dress) is made up entirely of pintucks, with lace insertions.

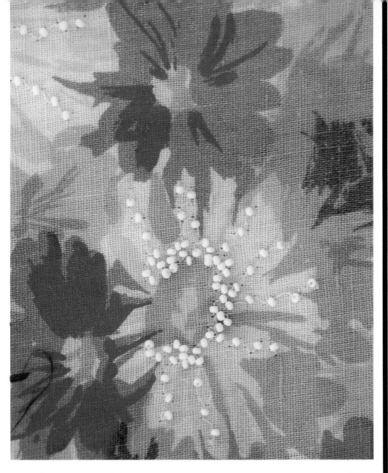

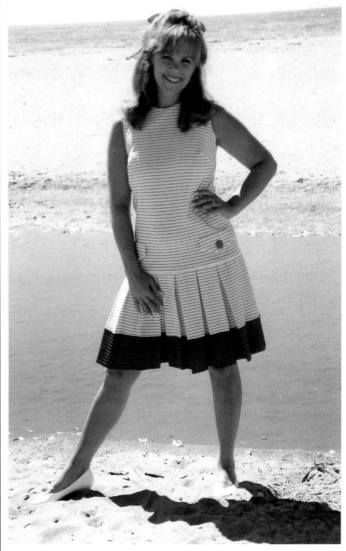

A nautical polyester sixties dress. *Courtesy of The Very Little Theatre.*

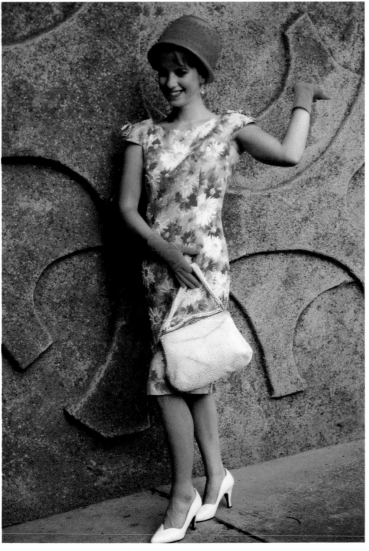

This fun, colorful, very sixties dress was home made and exceptionally sewn. The linen fabric is covered entirely with printed flowers, which are hand-embellished with periodic white beading.

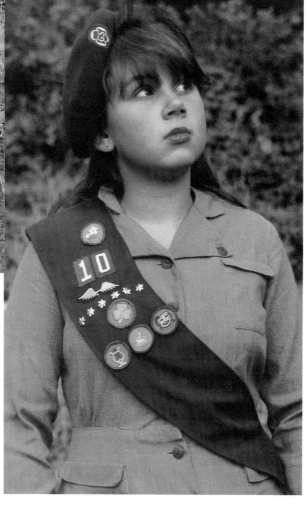

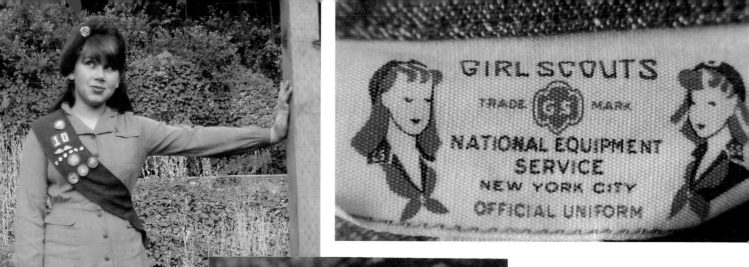

A complete Girl Scout's uniform: Dress, banner, and hat. *Courtesy of Flossy McGrew's.*

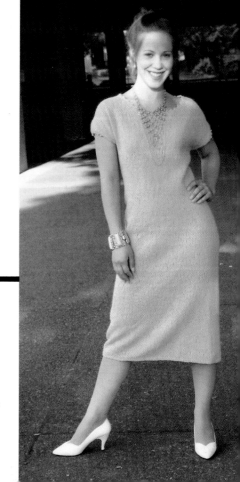

An easy, modern knit chemise dress with a matching jacket. *Courtesy of The Very Little Theatre.*

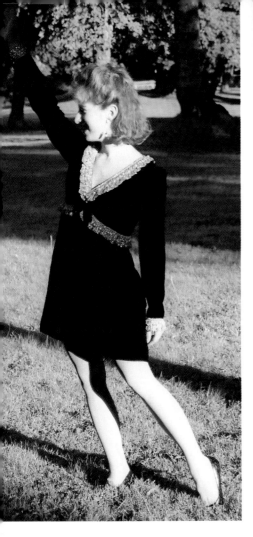

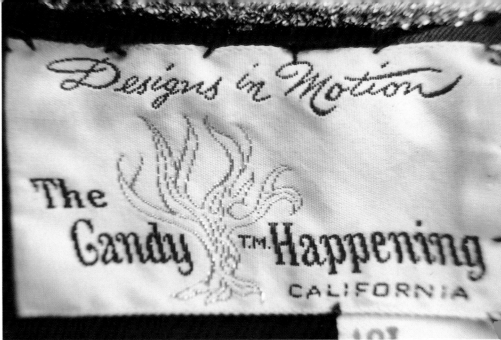

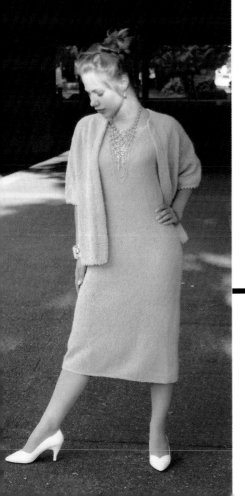

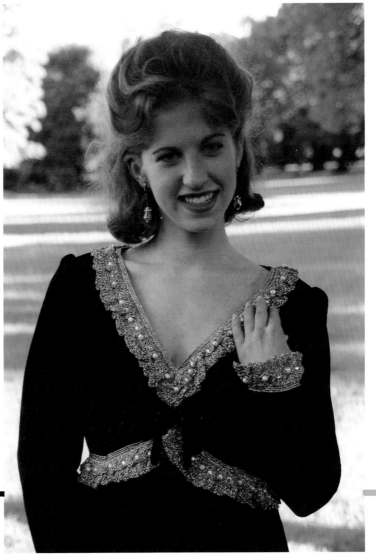

This "Designs in Motion" party dress of brown velvet is trimmed with typically-sixties metallic lace and features a plastic zipper running down its back. *Courtesy of Jerri Bickmore.*

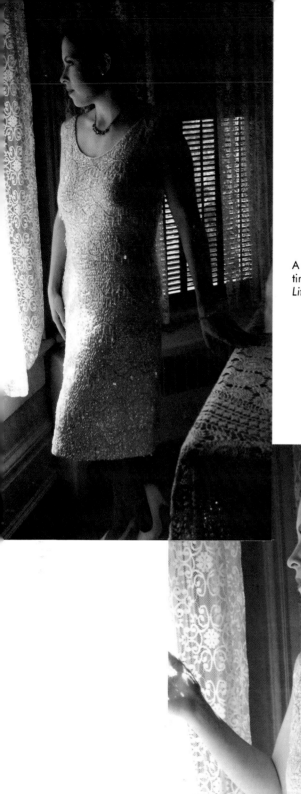

A delicate beaded chemise dress with
tiny beaded fringe. *Courtesy of The Very
Little Theatre.*

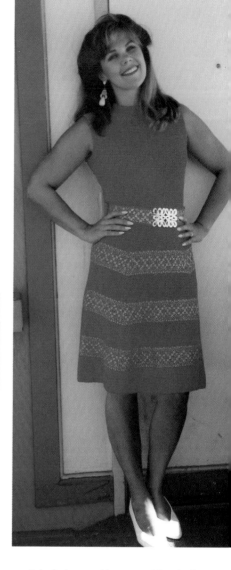

A knit dress with a matching belt.
Courtesy of The Very Little Theatre.

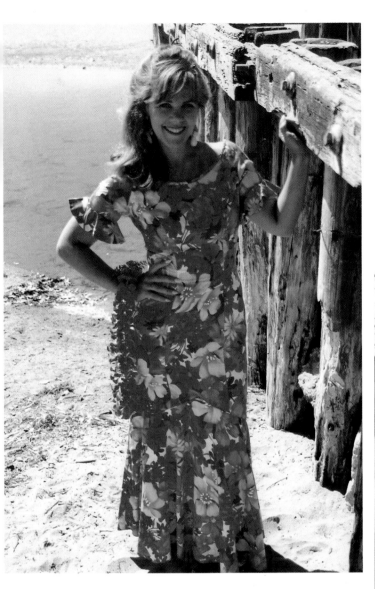

"There are no ugly women, only lazy ones."
- Helena Rubinstein, My Life for Beauty, 1966.

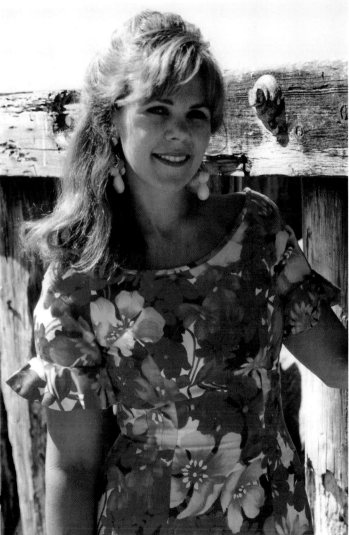

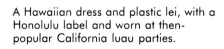

A Hawaiian dress and plastic lei, with a Honolulu label and worn at then-popular California luau parties.

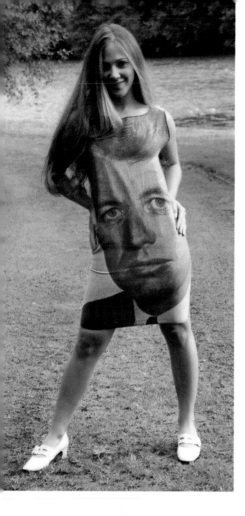

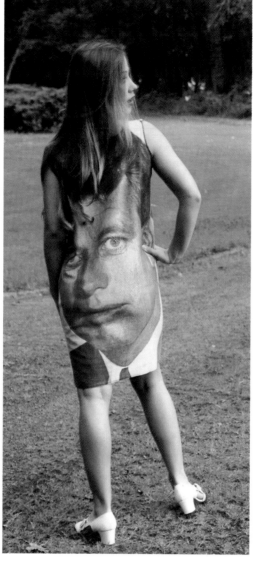

A remarkable knit tube dress made up with a single side seam. The original owner remembers this unusual dress was from John F. Kennedy's election campaign. *Courtesy of D. Lisa Rand.*

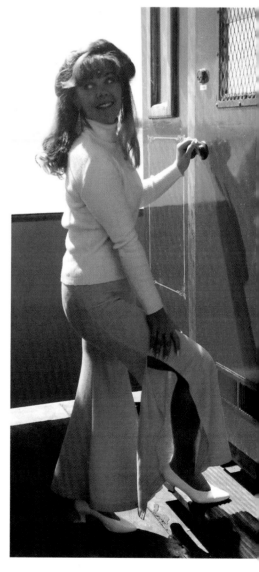

A late 1960s T-shirt. *Courtesy of D. Lisa Rand.*

These poly-knit bellbottoms with a long side slit were a favorite of their original owner, who wore them on casual occasions.

124

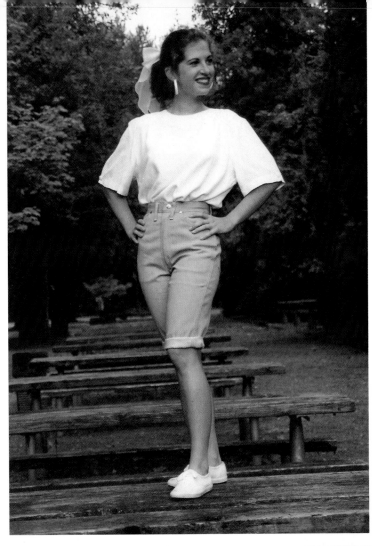

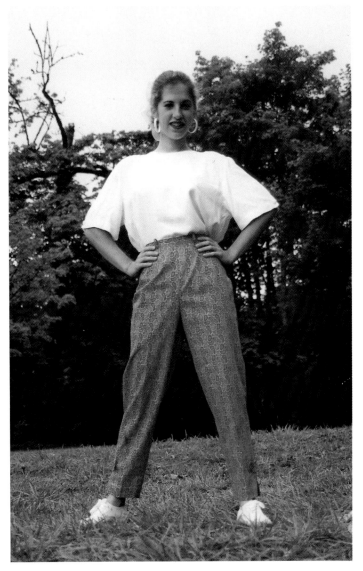

Cotton pants in a brilliant paisley fabric. *Courtesy of Flossy McGrew's.*

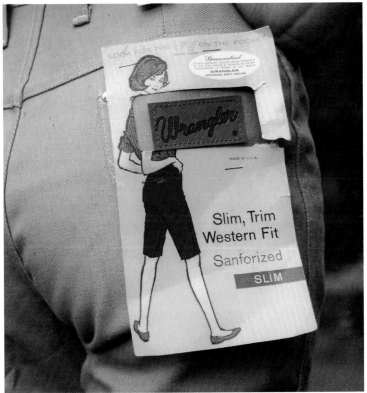

One might suspect these jean-shorts were brand new—except for the attached sales label, which clearly dates them to the 1960s. *Courtesy of Flossy McGrew's.*

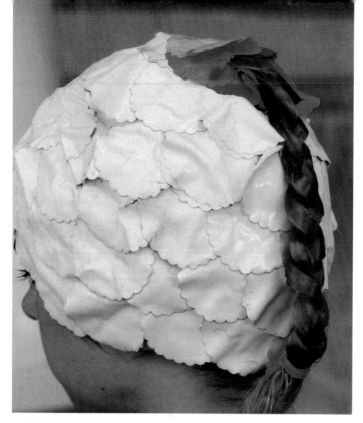

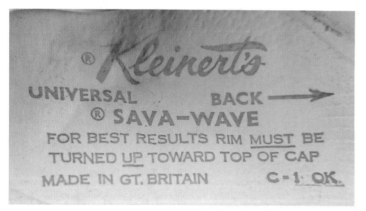

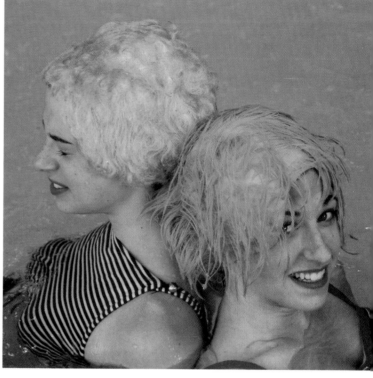

Funky bathing caps replaced silly sunglasses in the 1960s. This one features a hair braid falling from its crown and a Kleinert's label. *Courtesy of Flossy McGrew's.*

For the girl brave at heart, "hair" bathing caps. *Courtesy of Flossy McGrew's.*

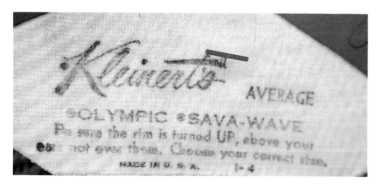

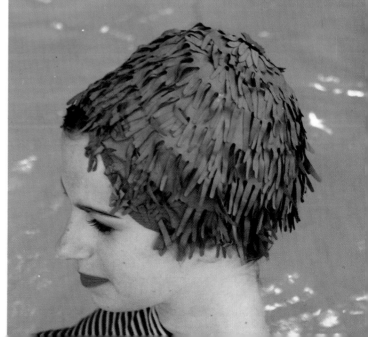

A Kleinert's "Olympic" bathing cap. *Courtesy of Flossy McGrew's.*

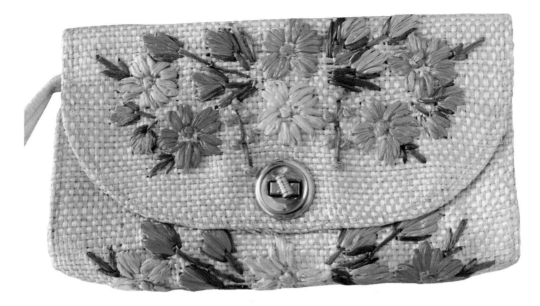

A typical sixties clutch.

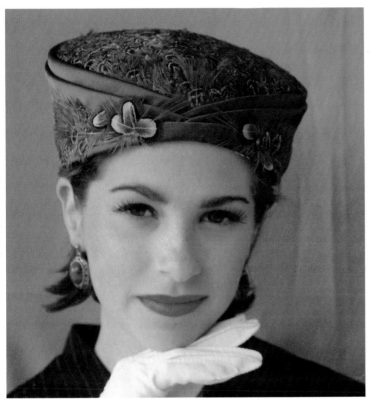

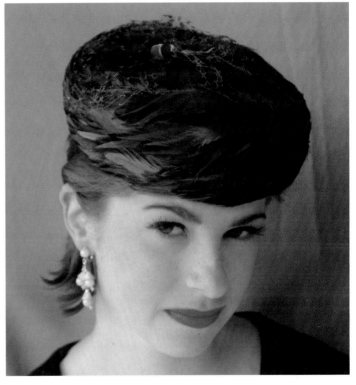

In shades of emerald and forest green, a delicate hat. *Courtesy of The Very Little Theatre.*

A truly chic hat with expert use of feathers. *Courtesy of The Very Little Theatre.*

127

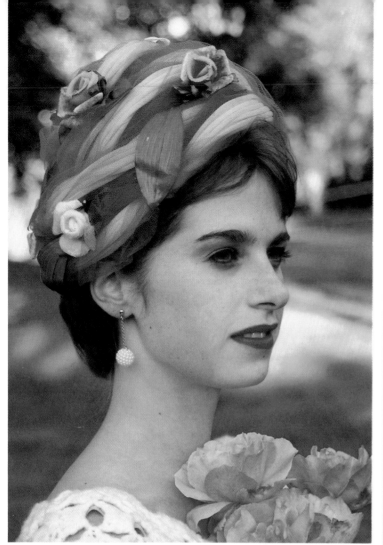

"Overaggression is certainly unfeminine, and although you may resort to it, I don't think you'll be very comfortable. True, your friends may make lengthy phone calls to boys; do all the party planning and inviting...But somehow, just as in business and in marriage, someone has to be the leader. And in a man-woman relationship, I doubt whether any woman can boss a real man."
- Seventeen, November 1957.

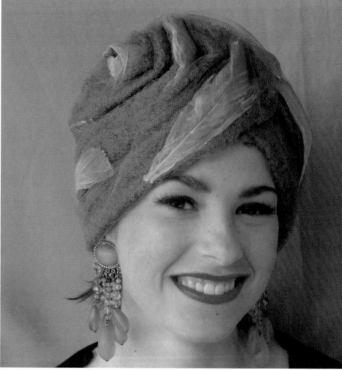

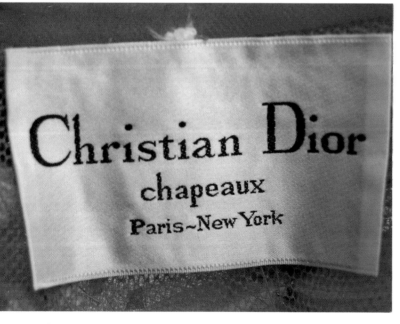

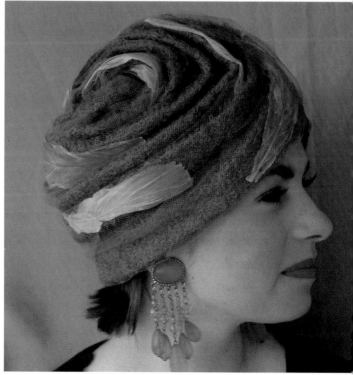

Two Christian Dior hats from the 1960s, each is in the turban-style. The green hat has feathers "floating" beneath an outerlayer of netting; the pink is blooming with faux roses. Green hat courtesy of *The Very Little Theatre*; pink hat courtesy of *Marianine's Vintage Chic*.

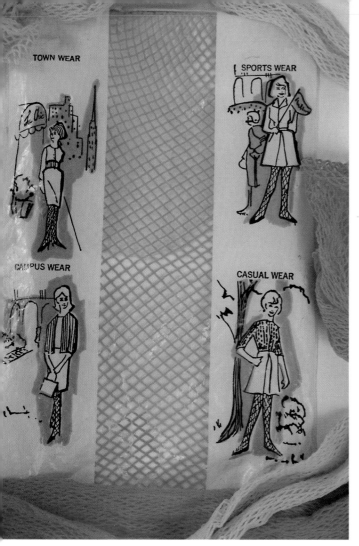

TOWN WEAR

SPORTS WEAR

CAMPUS WEAR

CASUAL WEAR

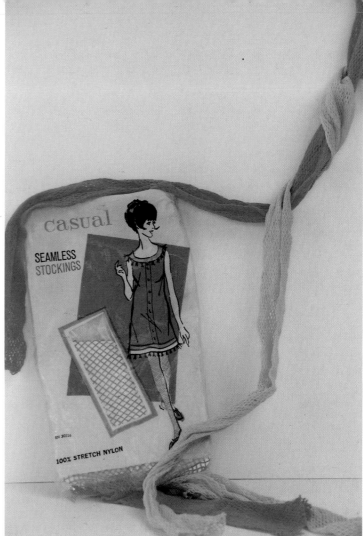

casual

SEAMLESS
STOCKINGS

100% STRETCH NYLON

Nylon fishnet stockings from the 1960s, in their original packaging. In the most trendy colors, these would have been worn by a hip young woman.

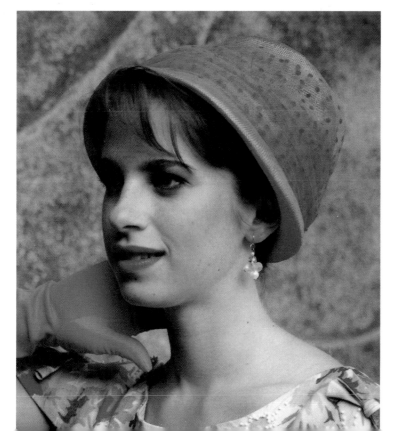

Orange was a highly popular color throughout the 1950s, and especially in the 1960s. This straw hat dates to the sixties and is embellished only with a band of fine netting. *Courtesy of The Very Little Theatre.*

A purse decorated with machine embroidery, covered by plastic. *Courtesy of The Very Little Theatre.*

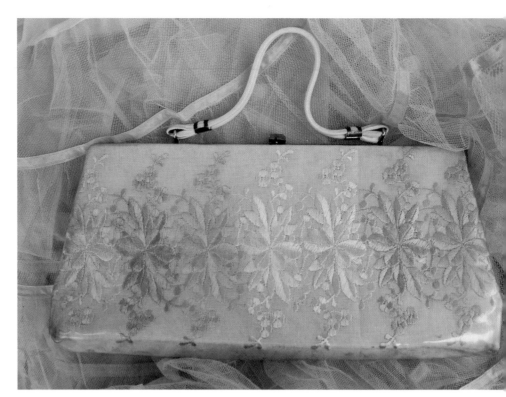

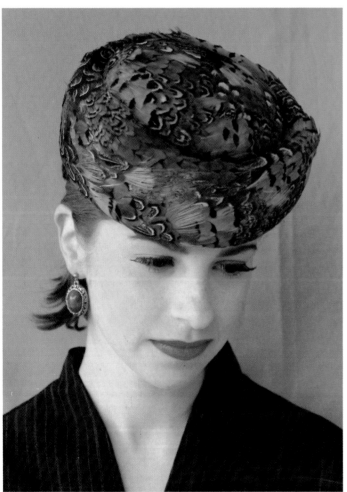

This classy burgundy feather hat is labeled "Oriental Millinery; Tokyo and Shanghai." *Courtesy of The Very Little Theatre.*

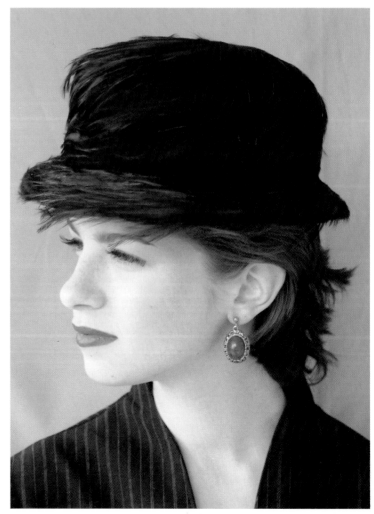

A sophisticated pillbox. *Courtesy of The Very Little Theatre.*

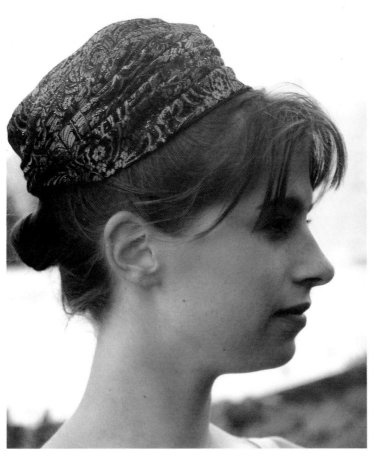

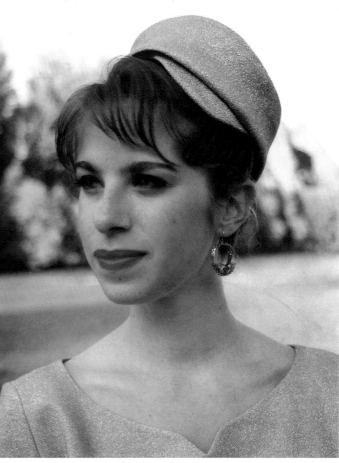

A metallic modified pillbox ideal for perching atop a big hairdo. *Courtesy of The Very Little Theatre.*

This soft pillbox of metallic-shot satin dates to the 1960s. *Courtesy of The Very Little Theatre.*

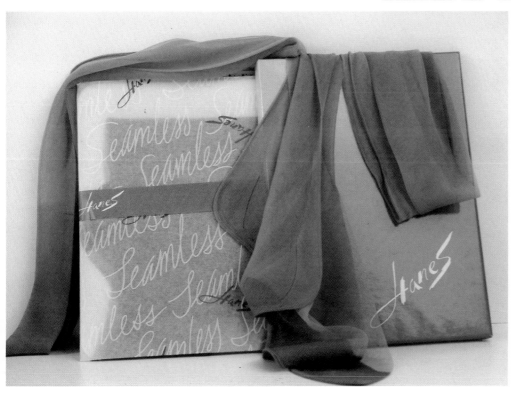

Hanes seamless stockings in their original packaging.

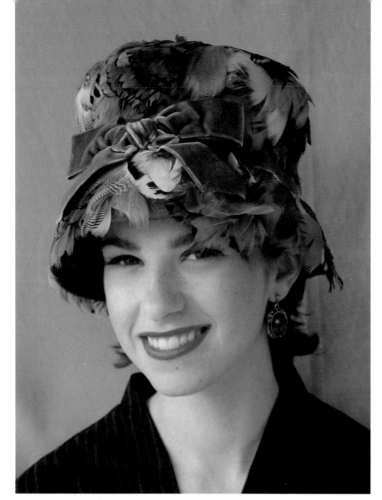

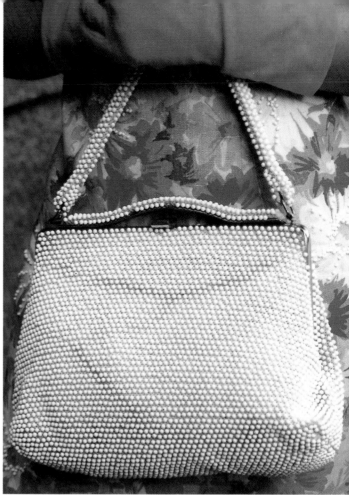

This 1960s purse features all over beading. *Courtesy of The Very Little Theatre.*

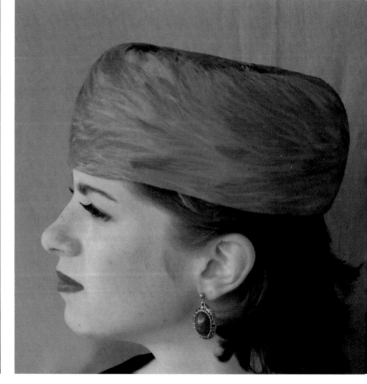

This coy sixties feather hat is set-off with the decade's hall-mark: a soft bow. *Courtesy of The Very Little Theatre.*

Small in size but brilliant in color, this little hat is a "Marché Exclusive." *Courtesy of The Very Little Theatre.*

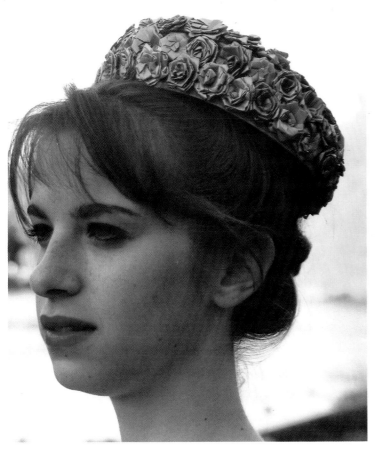

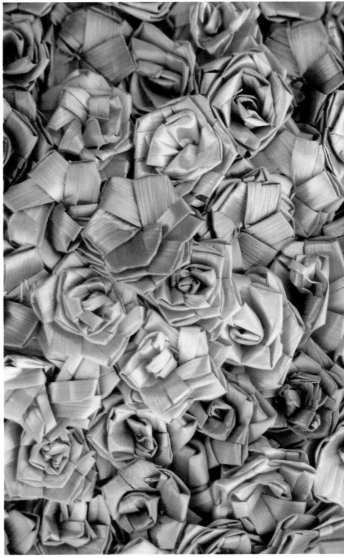

An unusual hat, this "I Magnin" pillbox is covered entirely with paper flowers. *Courtesy of The Very Little Theatre.*

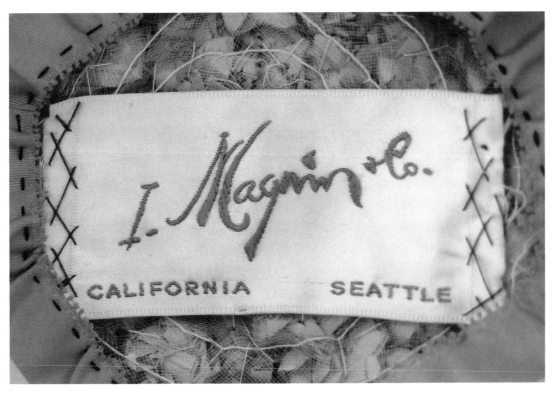

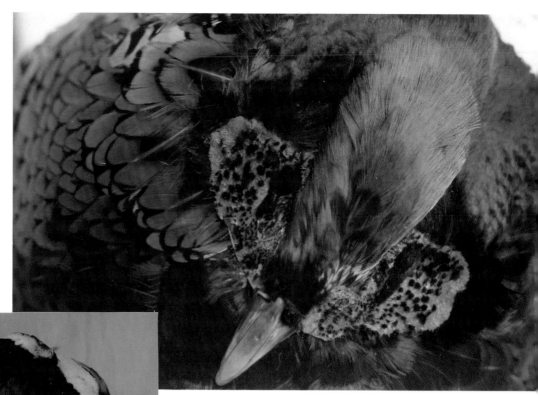

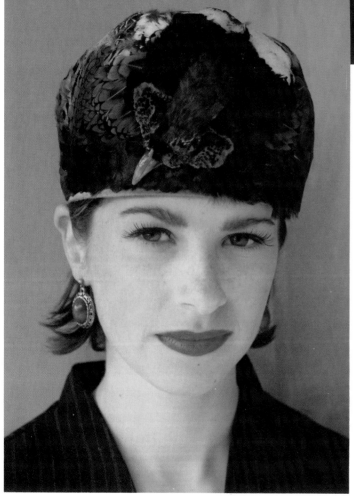

Custom made in the early 1960s, Martha Hichens created this hat from the feathers of a China pheasant shot by her grandson. *Courtesy of The Very Little Theatre.*

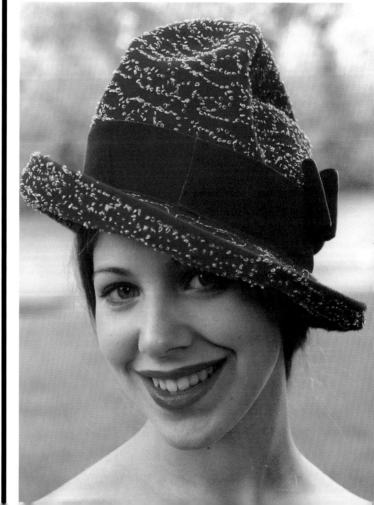

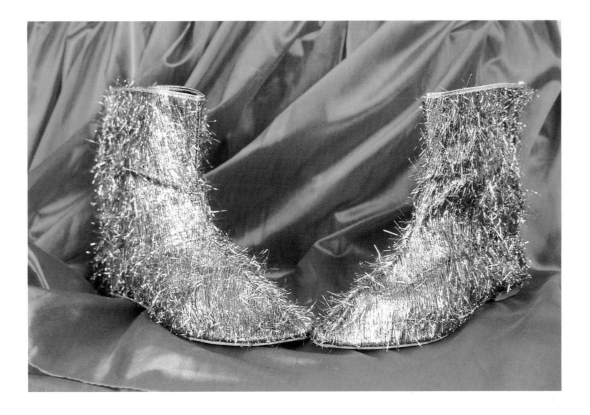

Funky gold tinsel boots from the 1960s made by "Bertlun of New York." *Courtesy of The Very Little Theatre.*

A young and trendy velvet hat from the late 1960s. *Courtesy of Flossy McGrew's.*

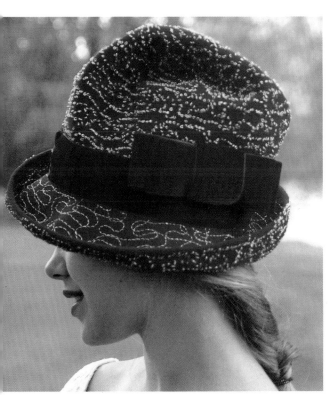

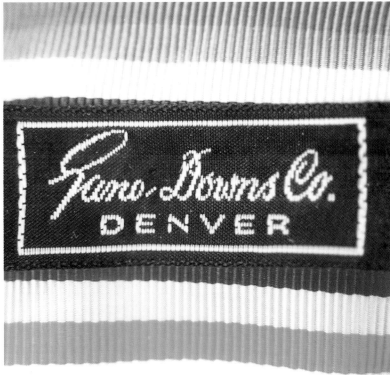

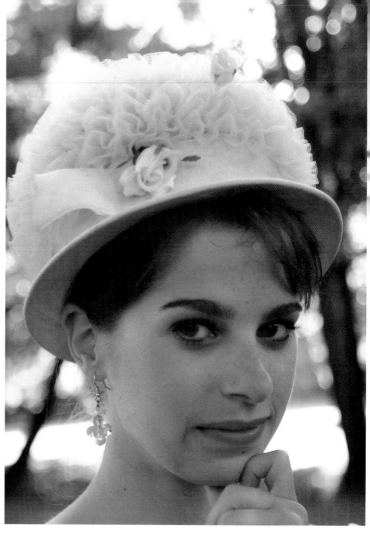

A beehive hat from the 1960s, whose crown is covered entirely with ruched netting. *Courtesy of The Very Little Theatre.*

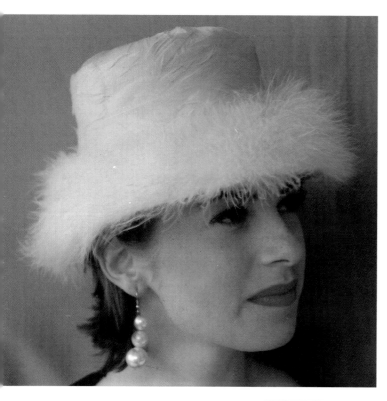

Two soft, feminine hats. The white hat is labeled "Happy Cappers, by the Field Company, Los Angeles, Ca." *Courtesy of The Very Little Theatre.*

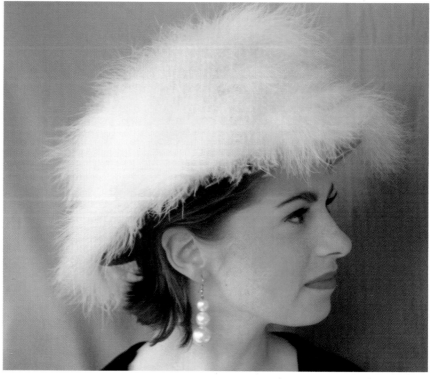

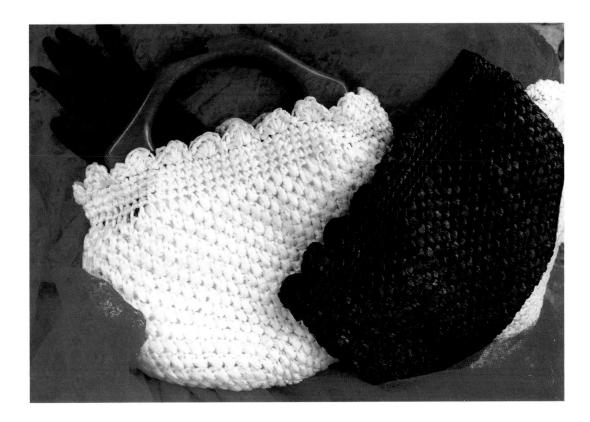

An everyday purse from the sixties with interchangeable crocheted bags of white, ecru, and black that can be buttoned onto its handle.

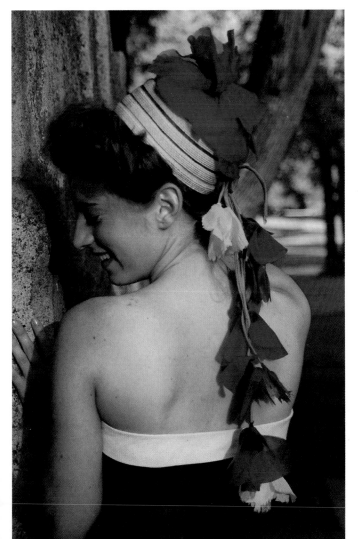

A natural straw hat made frivolous and fun with the addition of rayon poppies. The hat contains a "Miss Dior" label, indicating it was created for the youth market.

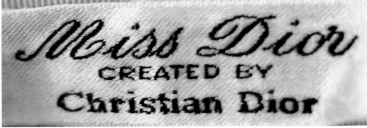

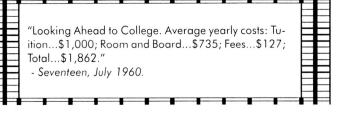

"Looking Ahead to College. Average yearly costs: Tuition...$1,000; Room and Board...$735; Fees...$127; Total...$1,862."
- *Seventeen, July 1960.*

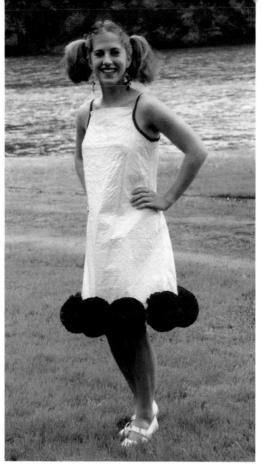

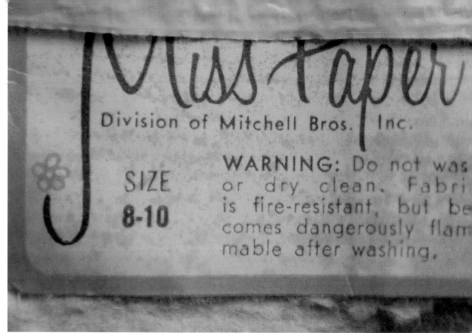

A paper party dress by Miss Paper; it is rather like a shower curtain and is in the "wipe-off" category of paper dresses. *Courtesy of Flossy McGrew's.*

The "Yellow Pages" paper dress. The original owner, Jerri Bickmore, recalls she purchased the dress in August of 1968 through an ad in *The Wall Street Journal* for $4. "I did wear it shopping a couple of times when it was new," Jerri says, "but decided that doing so could be embarrassing!" The dress feels rather like Pellon or dry, thick baby wipes. *Courtesy of Jerri Bickmore.*

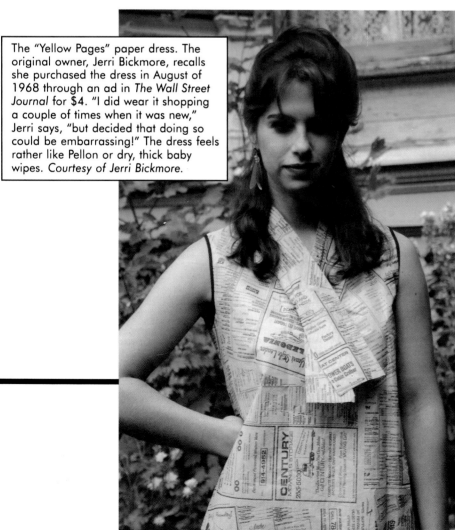

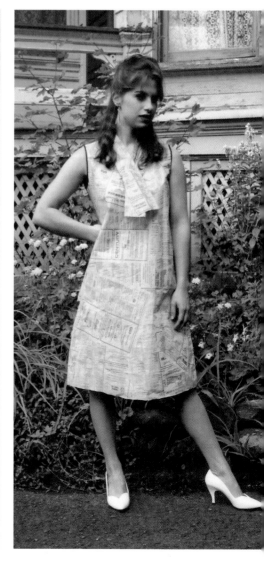

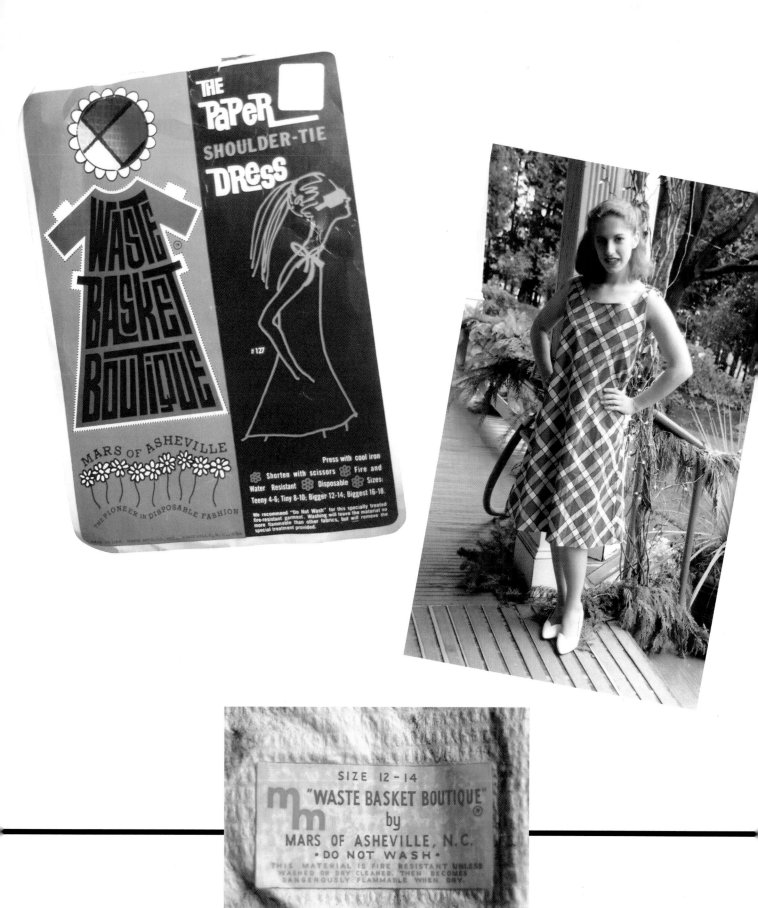

This colorful Mars of Asheville paper dress is still in its original plastic packaging. *Courtesy of Rose Ogden.*

To find a paper dress still in its original, untampered packing—as shown here—is unusual. *Courtesy of Klassic Line Vintage Clothing.*

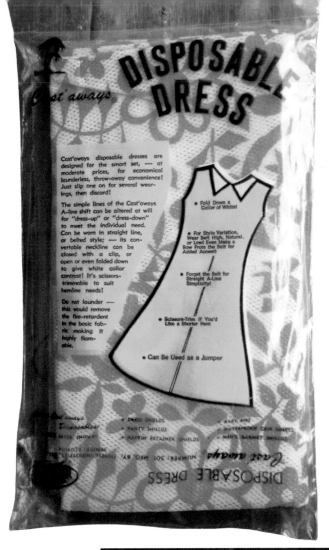

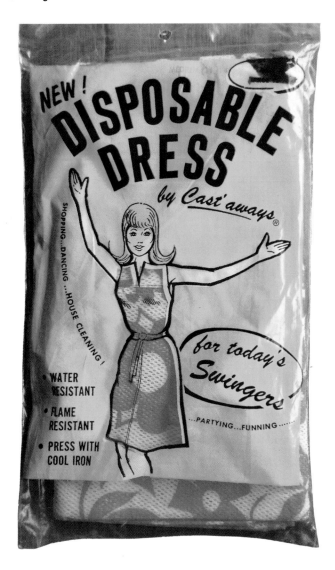

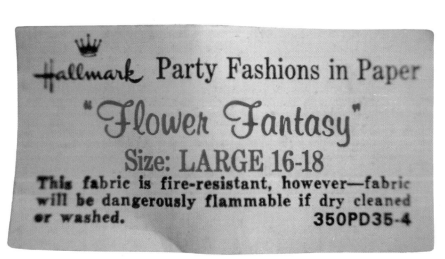

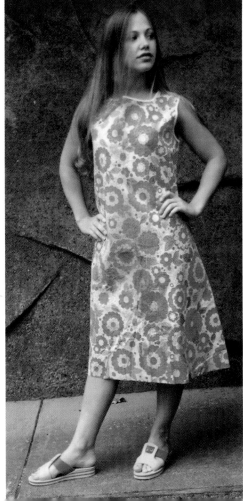

A Hallmark paper dress—which feels like its made of very strong crepe paper—worn with plastic "flip-flop" shoes. *Courtesy of Flossy McGrew's.*

...And Beyond

Though today fashions beyond the 1960s are not yet generally considered collectible, there is no doubt they soon will be. Certainly, now is the time to buy fashions from the 1970s forward; it is easier today to discover the finest examples at the least cost, making any inevitable increase in value a happy predictable. But the question is, just what will be considered collectible in the future?

As with anything else, the whims and fancies of collectors are impossible to predict precisely, but it seems to me there are three very different paths collectors can take on the road to future fashion collectibles. The most obvious is couture designer wear. Though not inexpensive to begin with, couture wear will always have a market—though it will probably be subject to the same ups and downs couture fashions have had in the collectibles field in the past. The second path is to collect the extraordinary fashions on the cutting edge of each decade—like the punk rock fashions of the eighties, for example; things that were rarely worn except by a select avant guard group. The third path is to collect styles worn by more "everyday" women.

Not only are the latter fashions more accessible to the majority of collectors, but they will also provide the sharpest picture of the women of the era—which, ultimately, is what collectible fashions are all about. In this vein then, what can we expect to become most desirable? I would imagine that good examples of the peasant and prairie looks of the 1970s will be desirable (especially by ready-to-wear designers Jessica McClintock—both her Gunne Sax label and her own house label—and Laura Ashley. McClintock and Ashley, it should be noted, are still designing today; no doubt their designs from the 1980s forward will also be collectible—though probably not as highly valued, since they vary from mainstream fashion and cling to the soft, Victorian-inspired look which was at the height of fashion in the Seventies.) From the Seventies, too, beautiful examples of African-inspired designs, and styles hinting at the fashions of the 1930s (inspired by the Warren Beatty, Faye Dunaway film *Bonnie and Clyde*) may also be sought after. "Hot Pants" and bell-bottoms will be sought by some, and as difficult to believe as it might be for those of us who remember them, polyester-knit pantsuits are already becoming favorites among young collectors.

From the 1980s, dresses inspired from the 1950s, with ballooning skirts held out by attached crinolines (a style that lasted into the early 1990s) will probably

be a collector's favorite, among the "power suits" and broad-shouldered dresses of the period. The eighties variation on the chemise dress, with a few flounces at the hem and fabric flowers or flounces at the shoulder, are a hallmark of the era, and good examples of this style may be valuable in the future. The basic evening dress of the eighties, with a moderately full, long skirt, fitted bodice, and ballooning sleeves will probably be relatively easy to find in the future, but exceptional examples will certainly be prized, just as slender, knee-length evening gowns with enormous, puffed sleeves will likely be. The most classy dresses and suits (the basic, slim black with large white collars and the red suit/dress with gold buttons and black collars and cuffs, for example), à la Princess Diana may also prove quite collectible, as may "bubble" dresses, whose skirts are gathered at both the top and bottom.

It has always been difficult for collectors and fashion historians to look at fashions from their own era with an unbiased eye, and so it may seem that fashions from the 1990s and into the 21st century are so

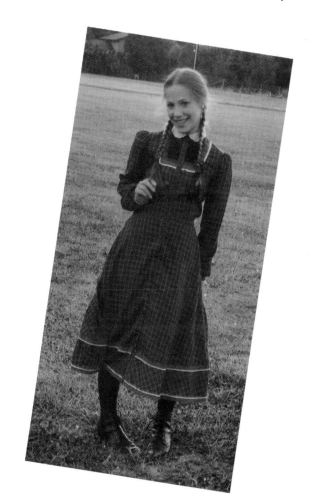

In the 1970s, the girlish "prairie" look came into fashion, headed by Jessica McClintock. *Courtesy of The Very Little Theatre.*

141

eclectic its impossible to pinpoint what trends will be most favored in the future. This may be true (though I'm inclined to believe that with proper perspective, major trends will become more obvious—like the thirties revival chiffon and rayon dresses of the mid-1990s). However, one thing at least you learn when you are a fashion collector: to look at your own clothing with new perspective. This includes an awareness of what—from your very own closet—might someday be a collector's item. Whenever I do my spring cleaning, sorting through everything from evening dresses to jeans in my closet, and I run across something I haven't worn in several years for one reason or another, I don't throw it out immediately the way fashion magazines and organization books tell you to. First, I stop and reflect on whether or not this dress (or sweater, or hat, or pair of shoes...whatever) might be collectible one day.

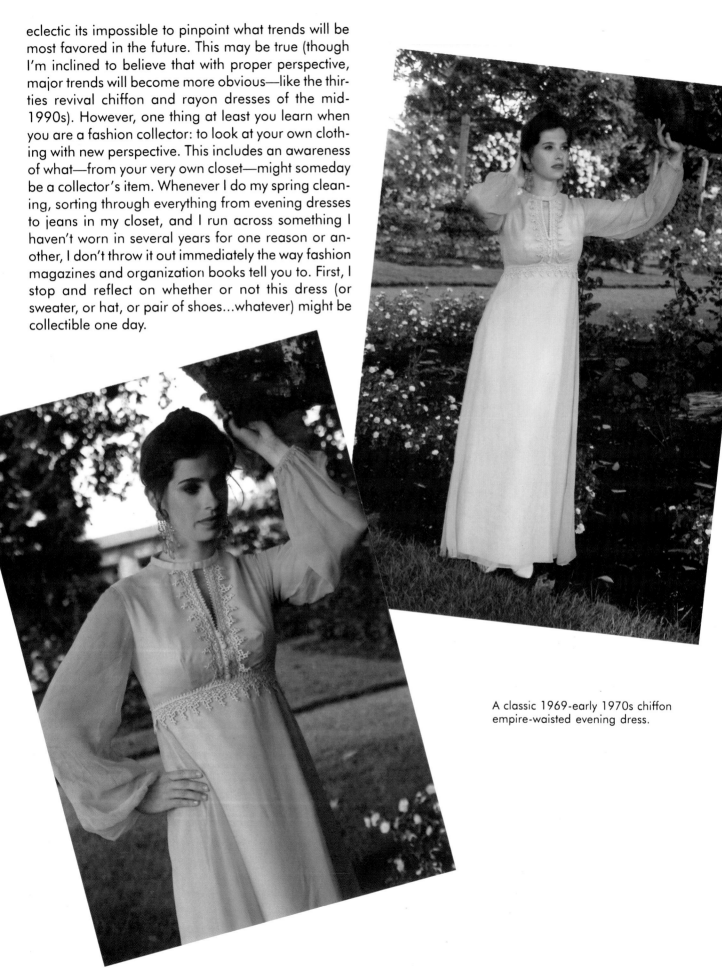

A classic 1969-early 1970s chiffon empire-waisted evening dress.

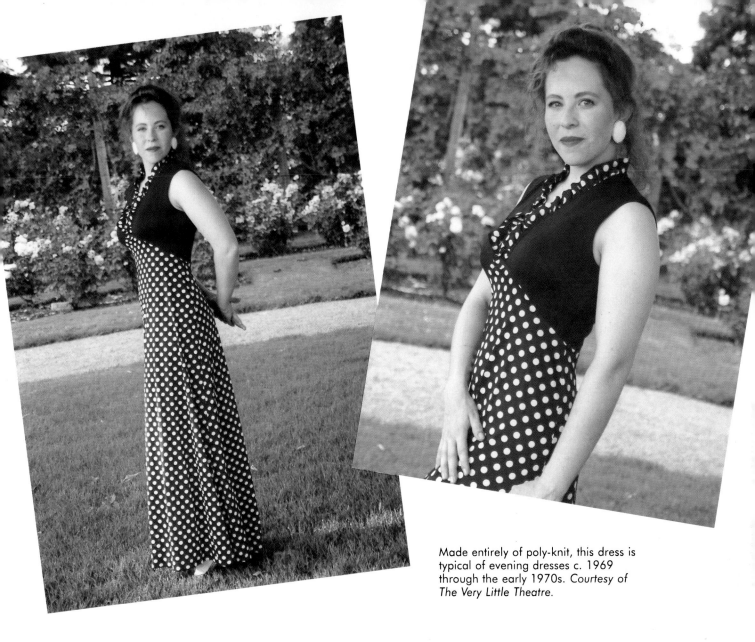

Made entirely of poly-knit, this dress is typical of evening dresses c. 1969 through the early 1970s. *Courtesy of The Very Little Theatre.*

By considering the condition of the piece (mint or excellent condition, preferably), the quality of the garment (reasonably well made—or, better yet, exceptionally made), and whether or not it typifies an era or trend, I may decide to hang on to the garment and tuck it away with my other fashion collectibles.

Of course, no one can say for certain what will be collectible in coming years. *National Geographic* magazine is a classic example of how the best planning can be undermined. When Americans saw this beautifully photographed, excellently written magazine, thousands of them decided not to throw away their issues—to keep them for the future, when certainly, they thought, they would be collectible and valuable. Unfortunately, so many people saved their *National Geographic*s that today they are so common they aren't worth a great deal. Someday you and I may find ourselves in a similar predicament; so many people may save Gunne Sax dresses, for example, that they will be so common they will hardly be worth

the attention of collectors. (Of course, give anything time and it may come around. Once black silk dresses from the turn of the century were so common that collectors largely ignored anything but the most exceptional examples. Today however, they are becoming more scarce, and have increased considerably in value. By the same token, sheer, white, lacy dresses from the same time period have always been available in abundance; this has not stopped their value from staying in the several hundred dollar range for excellent examples, however. Sometimes, despite an overflow of availability, the beauty of the garment wins out.)

All this may lead you to wonder: Isn't all this speculation risky? Not unless you're paying large sums for these relatively new fashions. But most fashions from the 1970s forward are available at thrift shops and garage sales for 50¢ to $20—and many will probably be free, from the closets of friends and family, or even your very own wardrobe.

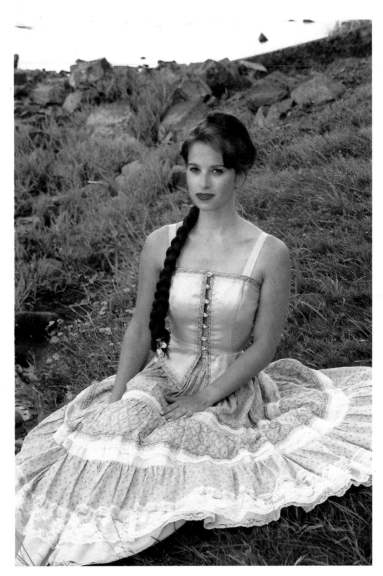
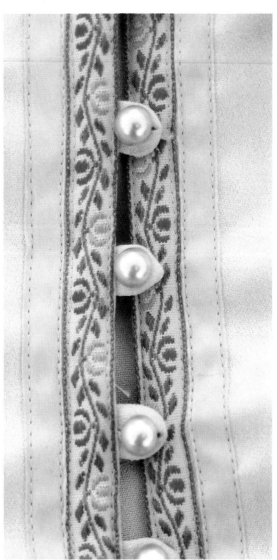
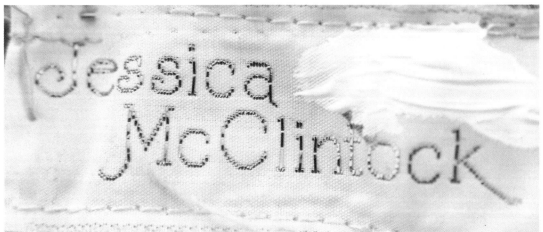

A Jessica McClintock dress from the 1970s, featuring a satin bodice with a peplum, and a cotton and satin layered skirt. *Courtesy of The Very Little Theatre.*

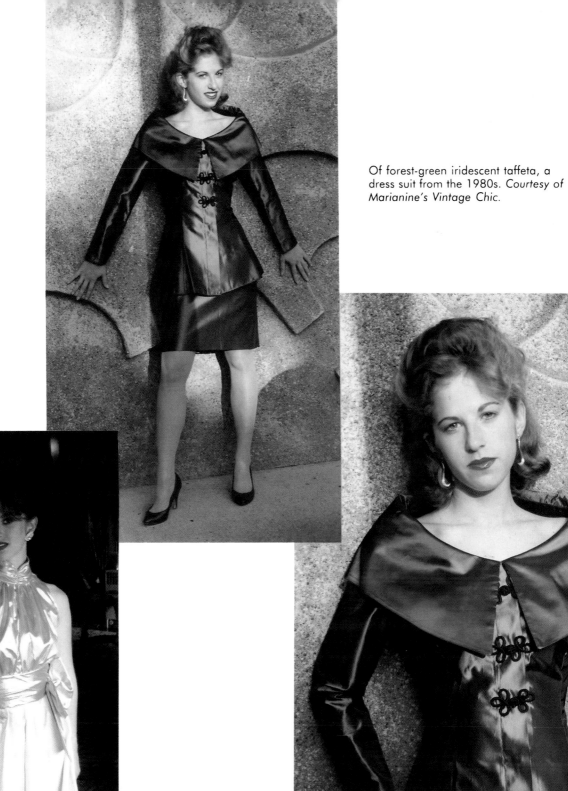

Of forest-green iridescent taffeta, a dress suit from the 1980s. *Courtesy of Marianine's Vintage Chic.*

A bubble dress and matching pumps from 1987, featuring a metallic bodice and a taffeta skirt with net crinoline beneath.

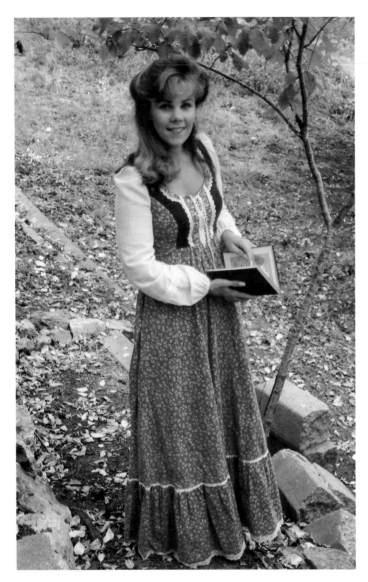

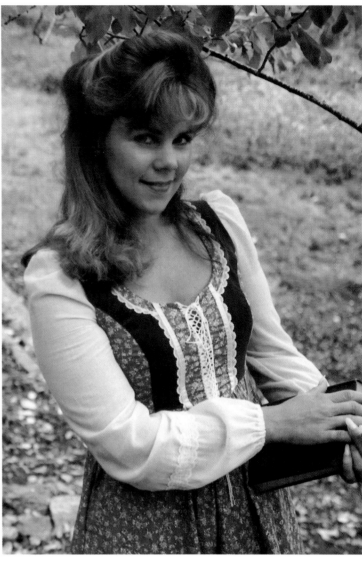

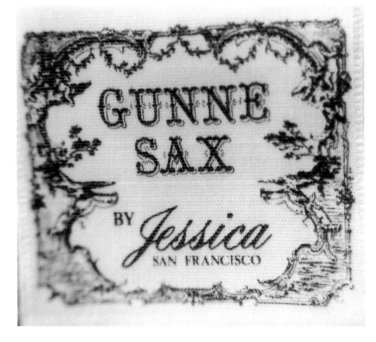

A charming 1970s Gunne Sax dress of calico, fine cotton, lace, satin ribbon, velvet, and a lace-up bodice.

PART TWO

The average woman of the 1950s-60s had a great deal more clothing than most women of any earlier era; this, coupled with the relative youth of fashions from this period, make the fashions of the fifties and sixties the easiest of all types of vintage clothing to find today. Too, because the fashions of this era are still inexpensive compared to earlier types of fashion collectibles, there are excellent opportunities to acquire fashions in the best condition and at the least amount of money. Unlike fashions from the 19th (or even the early 20th) century—where collectors often have to sacrifice acquiring the finest quality because of lack of funds—nearly every collector has the opportunity to purchase fine quality fashions from the 1950s forward.

Value & Provenance

Other benefits to collecting from this era abound—including the enhanced chance of obtaining provenance. Provenance—or the history behind a garment which can be traced directly to its original owner—can add as much as 50% to the value of any given item (depending upon how famous the person is you can trace it to), so it pays to do a little asking around whenever you acquire a piece. If you purchase something from a shop or show, always ask if the dealer knows anything about who the original owner of the garment was. Sometimes, armed with a name and (if you're lucky) a phone number, it is relatively easy to contact that person and find out more about the garment. But whether you acquire the piece from a dealer or from the original owner (or a relative of the original owner), whatever information you can discover about the garment itself should be put into writing. A simple note, signed and dated by the original owner or her descendant is extremely helpful. (The first being most desirable, since family members sometimes have faulty memories about the history behind their relative's garments.) If the garment was worn at a wedding, a confirmation, a graduation, or any other event, be certain this information is included. If there are recollections of choosing the fabric and having a local dressmaker stitch up the garment, note this too. If there are photographs of the original owner donning the garment, be certain to obtain a copy of some sort—preferably a photographic copy, though often a color laser copy is more practical.

Once you have this information in hand, tuck it away safely. A documentation book is extremely helpful for this purpose—and a great "show-off" book besides! Mine is simply a binder with sheets of paper kept inside plastic protectors. Here, I log all my acquisitions by storing sales receipts, photographs of every item in my collection, any information I have on the provenance of each piece, and brief descriptions of every item. Not only is this a great way to keep track of where my collection is headed, but it's ideal for both appraisal and insurance purposes. (For pieces with provenance, I also store the note given to me by the original owner in my brag book, while keeping a copy of it with the actual garment.)

While it may seem that you could just as easily store all this information in your head, the truth is our memories are often faulty; and when someday someone else acquires the garment, they will have no idea of the true provenance of the piece unless you keep that information accessible and on paper. Too, true provenance—the kind that can add value to your collection—only comes with written documentation from the original owner or her descendant. (It is no coincidence the word is spelled P-R-O-V-E-N-ance!)

Value & Condition

Condition is all when it comes to collectible fashions—and clothing from the 1950s-60s are expected to be in especially great shape. Tears, holes, and stains are not acceptable to most collectors, since there are still far too many excellent-condition garments from this era available. In order to keep your collection in excellent condition, retain its value, and allow it to increase in value over the years, a little attention to care should be paid.

Fashions from the fifties and sixties are easily attended to, and care is mostly a matter of common sense. It is best if clothes are stored flat (hangers—even padded ones—strain shoulder- and waist-lines, eventually causing excess wear in those areas). Some collectors prefer to store garments in chests of drawers, but many find cardboard boxes more suitable for larger collections. Either way, every drawer or box should be lined with an old white sheet (white because a colored sheet may eventually stain garments resting against it) or muslin fabric. This keeps the acids found in wood and cardboard from eating away at the fabrics in your collection. Tissue should be used to pad folds, decreasing the chances of permanent wrinkles or fold-lines appearing; however, only acid-free tissue (available at art supply stores) should be used, since regular tissue paper contains acids that will eventually cause yellow spots on fabric. If the garment is made of silk, only a white sheet or muslin fabric should be used to pad it; silk has a tendency to be weaker than any other type of fabric, and the fewer folds you use in storing it, the better.

Plastic bags suffocate clothing—literally. Fabrics need to be able to breathe in order to say in good condition. Plastic bags seal in moisture, and don't allow air to circulate around the garment, eventually causing mildew and mold. If you want extra protection for special garments (especially those which are beaded or have lace trimmings that might catch on other garments' zippers, buttons, or hooks and eyes), use a white fabric bag in place of plastic.

Some items from the sixties and Seventies are also made of polyvinyl chloride (PVC) and require extra attention. PVC gives off a chlorine gas, which is harmful to fabrics; therefore, any item made of PVC should be stored in a separate box, and, preferably, in a separate location.

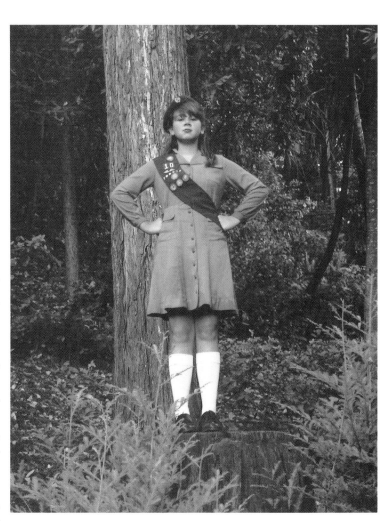

Collectors of fashions from the 1950s onward have unsurpassed opportunities to uncover garments with recordable history behind them.

"Turn about is gay play with Velcro® nylon tape fastener...You just press Velcro® to close (it holds and holds!)—peel Velcro® to open. No ties, no buttons—and Velcro® is completely adjustable. Velcro® is as easy to sew as a simple seam. It can be washed, ironed, dry cleaned, cut to size...available at notions counters of leading stores in 11 fashion colors."
- Velcro ad, McCall's Pattern Fashions, 1960.

Furs are another special consideration for collectors. Never were furs more available to the average woman than in the 1950s; but real furs are difficult to store well. Most furs will only last about fifty years. To keep any furs (or garments trimmed with real fur) in the best condition for the longest period possible, store them in a cool place, separate from other garments. Place moth balls in the storage area (herbal mothballs are available which work well and do not have the pungent odor of traditional moth balls); cedar chips will also help keep pests away.

Because of the variety of materials paper dresses were created from, there are few hard-fast rules on caring for them. The most important thing to remember is that paper dresses and accessories were not intended to last any real length of time—they were meant to be disposable. Because of this, small tears or stains might be a little more acceptable to collectors—but any tears or stains that are noticeable and distracting *will* devalue the garment. One of the worst things you can do with a paper dress is try to remove a stain from it. It won't work and you're likely to rip the dress. The next worst thing you can do is try to repair a tear. Again, any repairs will only devalue the garment further, so it's best to leave it as is.

If the paper dress is considerably rumpled or has deep fold lines, it can be ironed—very carefully. Use a cool iron (no steam!) and test the effect on an inconspicuous spot. The best storage for a paper dress is probably to place it inside a stiff archival-quality poster envelope. This will keep it flat and protect it from ripping. If your storage space is limited and it's impossible to store such a large envelope, you might consider framing the dress. (Just be certain to use acid-free mountings and ultra-violet proof Plexiglass; then, hang it where direct sunlight will never reach it.) When all else fails, store paper fashions as flat as possible. Paper hats, shoes, and other accessories can be stored just like regular accessories, but each should be kept in their own separate box. Dresses, too, should be stored separate from fabric garments (some paper dresses may contain enough wood acids in them to cause yellow spots on fabric). It is definitely preferable for paper garments to be stored with as few folds as possible, but if some folds are necessary, pad them with rolled unbleached muslin, to prevent permanent creases.

Since it can be a risky undertaking, its best not to clean collectible clothing unless it is noticeably dirty. If this occurs, following the care and content label sewn into the garment is best. If, however, the garment contains no such label, a little caution is warranted. Fabrics new and varied were tried and experimented with during the 20th century; in the fifties, in particular, crease proof, wrinkle proof, stain proof, water proof, shrink proof, moth proof, and many others were used. Most of these experimentations were an attempt to make un-washable clothing washable. Nylon, for example, replaced rayon in most under-fashions and some outer-fashions. When in doubt, it is best to dry clean the garment. Still, dry cleaning does tend to make fabric brittle over time, and may yellow certain types of fabrics (one dealer even told me she took a couture designer garment of which she was exceedingly proud to a dry cleaner, only to pick it up the next day and discover it had fallen to pieces).

Garments which were originally intended to be washed in water should be handwashed (some sweaters were even created so they could be washed, then dried without blocking them). In order to keep the garment in its best condition, however, don't use your usual detergent. Even products marketed as "gentle," are really quite harsh on old fabrics. A little Neutrogena face wash soap works very well and is what the Smithsonian Institute uses on many of their textiles. (Use about 1/8 of a 3.5 oz. bar mixed with one cup of water, and add this to every gallon of washing water.) Gentle agitation is all that's needed (no squeezing or twisting), and soaking for no longer than twenty minutes is all that's necessary. The garment is then preferably dried on a sweater screen, which will prevent it from stretching or straining against a hanger or clothes line. Electric dryers are best avoided, as they tend to set stains (and may actually shrink fabrics which might not have ever been inside a dryer).

There is at least one last consideration when it comes to value and condition: Should you wear vintage clothing? Most museum experts will answer unequivocally: No. The reason for this is that fabrics are always more fragile than they appear (they are, after all, usually made up entirely or partially of plants; and you wouldn't expect a leaf to last 100—or even ten—years, would you?). Wearing vintage clothing puts that clothing into much greater risk of damage by rips, tears, holes, and staining. However, many collectors are satisfied that clothing from the 1950s-60s is sufficiently sturdy to be worn—at least on occasion. The decision is ultimately up to the individual collector; however, if you wish to keep your collection in tip-top condition, make it last for future generations, and continue to increase in value, its advisable not to wear it. Instead, many collectors opt to display their collections at local museums or historic homes—or even in their own homes. Just remember to keep textiles out of direct sunlight, and always let them breathe.

Value & Labels

Labels are not a means to an end. Collectors should not fall into the trap of thinking that a certain label will make a garment suddenly more valuable. While some people will only collect fashions with couture designer labels, for instance, this can be a risky investment. One year, designs by Chanel will skyrocket and sell for astronomical prices at the major auction houses. The next year, another designer may be "hot," and in time, that Chanel garment will not be valued at as much as was paid for it.

Too, labels can be misleading. Couture designer labels are sometimes sewn into non-couture clothing by unscrupulous sellers. Though sometimes it is immediately apparent that this has been done (because the garment is made with inferior construction), often the only clue that the garment might be authentic is that it contains a few couture hallmarks (like hand-finished seams or hand or bound buttonholes). However, since any of these hallmarks might be produced by an unknown dressmaker, this is hardly positive proof that you are, indeed, buying what the label claims you're buying.

There is also a *profound* difference between a custom couture garment (that is, a garment specifically stitched up for a particular client) and one that was created for the ready-to-wear market. Obviously, there is more of the latter, and these usually don't consist of the same fine quality that a custom couture garment (or perhaps even a garment created by a local dressmaker) does. A couture ready-to-wear garment is, understandably, less valued than a custom couture garment.

Since quality and beauty are utmost considerations when it comes to the value of fashions, a non-couture designer garment mass-produced and sold in thousands of local dress shops and department stores, or a garment made at home, or one created by a local dressmaker, can also be valued highly. Besides, one of the most fascinating things about collectible clothing is that it tells us so much about our history. In this respect, fashions worn by the masses—not created by couture designers—have the most historical significance.

Bearing all these things in mind, most collectors select a garment for their collection based upon its own merit. If a famous ready-to-wear designer or couture designer name happens to show up, its merely a pleasant surprise. Still, it is interesting to learn about the designers of any given era—both couture and non-couture. While a great deal has been written about couture designers, never have the ready-to-wear designers who clothed millions been acknowledged or documented.

What follows is an attempt to remedy this—a comprehensive list of designers well within the reach of the average collector—and the average woman of the 1950s-60s. The names listed are those that continually showed up either in the garments photographed in this book, or in middle-class fashion magazines of the era. Whenever possible, prices included in magazine copy or in manufacturer ads are included, along with dates from those sources.

When searching for labels on garments in your own collection, it is sometimes necessary to explore the interior of the garment entirely. Unlike most modern clothes, whose labels are almost always attached to the neck- or waist-line, many fashions from the 1950s-60s feature labels sewn under the arm, under attached crinolines, and even along side seams of skirts.

Other labels may be found throughout the book; consult the Index.

Ready-To-Wear Labels, Designers, & Manufacturers

Abraham & Straus
Paper clothes in the 1960s.
Accent
Shoes. (Example: $8.95-$11 in 1950.)
Adele Simpson
Moderately priced to expensive clothing. Opened in 1959; sold to 450 exclusive stores by 1967. Mrs. Lydon Johnson often wore Adele Simpson designs. The line was best known for careful attention to fine fabrics.

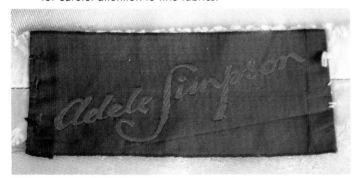

Aileen
Inexpensive clothing. (Example: day dress for about $12 in 1959.)
Aladdin
Inexpensive clothing. (Example: day dress for $3.95 in 1956.)
Alba
Stockings.
Alex Coleman
Inexpensive clothing. (Example: day dress for $13 in 1955.)

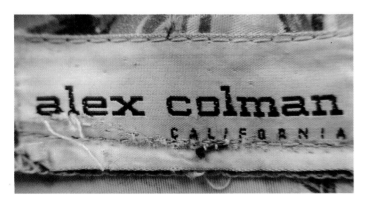

Andrew Arkin
Moderately priced clothing. (Example: suit for $40 in 1953.)
Anne Fogarty
Fogarty began as a designer for Youth Guild Inc.; in 1950, she left this manufacturer and joined Margot Dresses Inc. (dresses in the moderate range); in 1957, she went to Saks Fifth Avenue; she always received credit for her designs on labels (though some of her early Youth Guild designs were anonymous). In 1962, Fogarty created her own house, which sold to about 600 stores; dresses began at about $60.

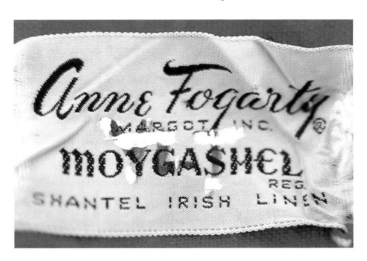

Annis
Inexpensive clothing. (Example: playsuit for $10 in 1955.)
Aptitudes
Shoes. (Example: $7.95 in 1953.)
Arnold & Fox
Moderately priced clothing. (Example: day dress for $35 in 1955; evening dress for about $65 in 1958.)
Arthur Jablow
Aywon Originals
Moderately priced clothing. (Example: skirt for $39.95 and day dress for $35 in 1952.)
Bali
Undergarments. (Ads found as early as 1952.)
Bally
Shoes.
Bare-Foot Originals
Shoes. (Example: $13 in 1958.)
Barra
Bags.
Bedford
Inexpensive clothing. (Example: day dress for $23 in 1950.)
Bell-Sharmeer
Stockings.
Ben Barrack
Moderately priced clothing. (Example: day dress for $39.95 in 1949.)
Berkshire
Stockings.
Bestform
Underfashions. (Example: $1.50-$5 in 1950.)
Betmar
Hats.
Betty Barclay
Inexpensive clothing. (Example: day dress for about $11 in 1955; day dress for about $15 in 1957.)

Betty Lane

Inexpensive clothing. (Example: day dress for about $25 in 1959.)

Bienen-Davis

Bags.

Bobby Brooks

Inexpensive clothing. (Example: day dress for $10 in 1967.)

Bobby Burns

Moderately priced clothing. "Figure Flattery for the 'In-Between.' "

Bonwit Teller

Moderately priced to expensive clothes. (Example: day dress for dress $49.95 in 1955; Suit $225 in 1955; day dress for $175 in 1955; day dress for $49.95 in 1955; bag for $12.95 in 1955) Also sold paper clothes in the late 1960s.

Braunstein's

Inexpensive clothing, particularly popular among young women. 1959 advertisement: "First he sees my jumper in a gay check [either red/white, lilac/white, or turquoise/white]...Next, its a lush [solid-color] rayon linen...then! I take off the suspenders and it becomes a skirt...has a special blouse all its own with checked collar and cuff to match. $8.95." (Example: day dress for $8.95 and blouse for $2.95 in 1957.)

Brigance of Sportmaker

Moderately priced clothes. (Example: blouse & skirt for about $25 each in 1955.)

Brilliant Sportswear

Bathing suits. (Example: $8-$11 in 1955.)

British Walkers

Shoes.

Bropar

Bags of handtooled leather, imported from Guatamal. (Example: $9.65 in 1953.)

Cabana

Inexpensive clothes. (Example: day dress for about $11 in 1950; bathingsuit for $17 in 1955.)

Cameo

Stockings; 1953 advertisement: "'Keep that soft misty glamour right down to your toes,' says Ava Gardner. Ava Gardner and dozens of other M-G-M stars know that shiny stockings pick up ugly highlights, make lovely legs look unshapely. That's why M-G-M stars wear Bur-Mil Cameo stockings on the screen and off. Cameo's exclusive Face Powder Finish glamourizes their legs with a permanently soft, misty dullness." From $1.15. In 1959, "seamed or seamless" styles advertised as available.

Cannon

Stockings; 1955 advertisement: "You don't know how wonderful stretch stockings can be until you wear Cannon stretch sheers."

Capezio

Shoes; Capezio began in 1887 as a maker of shoes for dancers. In 1944 they started making pumps based upon the general style of ballet slippers, which remained popular through the 1960s. Today Capezio has reverted to only manufacturing shoes for dancers and actors.

Caressa

Shoes. (Example: $16 in 1958.)

Carol King

Inexpensive clothing. (Example: party dress for about $25 in 1957; day dress for $18 in 1959.)

Carol Rodgers

Inexpensive clothing. (Example: day dress for about $13 in 1955; day dress for about $10 in 1960.)

Carolyn Schnurer

Inexpensive to moderately priced clothes. (Example: day dress for about $25 in 1950; day dress for about $40 in 1953; playsuit—on the cover of "Charm" fashion magazine—for $25 in 1955.)

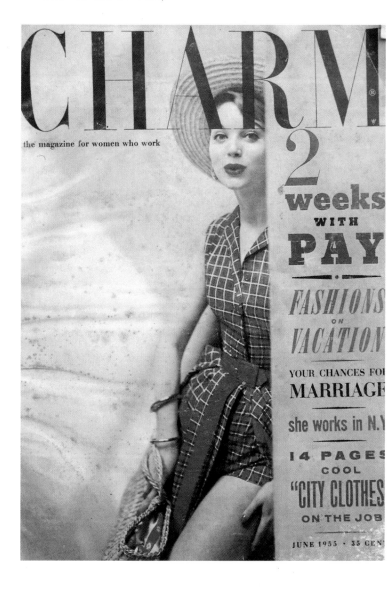

Catalina

Bathing suits; 1955 advertisement: "Lovely things happen to you in a Catalina. If you'd like to see a man thoroughly bewitched take a look at the next young man who takes a look at you in your Catalina swimsuit! Catalina designs this year feature such fashion innovations as the high rounded bosom and new lengthened torso. Catalina swimsuits also enhance your figure. (That's the famous Catalina knack of making swimsuits flatter different figure types.)" $11-19.95.

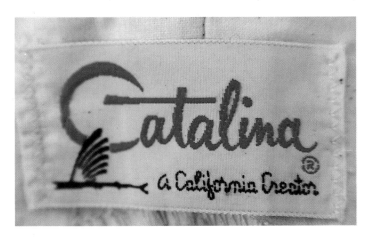

Cavanagh's

Inexpensive clothes. (Example: blouse for $8.50 in 1955.)

Ceil Chapman

Expensive clothes.

Charles Hymen

Inexpensive clothes. (Example: day dress for about $17 in 1955.)

Charles Sorel

Moderately priced clothes. (Example: day dress for $49 in 1949.)

Ciro

Inexpensive clothes. (Example: day dress for about $18 in 1950.)

Clair McCardell

McCardle began designing in the 1920s, and designing under her own label in 1940 for Towney Frocks. (Example: day dress for about $40 in 1955.)

Clayton Mfg. Co.

Plastic hoopskirts in the 1950s. Based in Atlanta, Georgia, the company's first ad appeared in a 1949 issue of "Glamour": "Belle-o-the-Ball COLLAPSIBLE Plastic Skirt Hoops. Adjusts to any size and figure, including "BUSTLE" and "FARTHINGALE" effects. Opens to a 90-inch skirt—folds to only 8 inches for packing and easy traveling. Light-weight, washable plastic—unlimited guarantee. The Belle-o-the-Ball Skirt Hoop is the modern essential to every college and bridal wardrobe. Perfectly balanced to support heavy materials and adds flattering poise to every formal. COMPLETE with rich plastic carrying case that doubles as extra make-up kit with handy compartment for accessories. At better stores or order direct. $14.50." Though it might seem that few women would wear such a hoopskirt when more modern crinolines (even full-length for evening wear) were available, the product was advertised too frequently in fashion magazines of the 1950s for it not to be popular.

Coblentz

Bags.

Cole of California

Inexpensive clothing. Advertisement for bathing suits in 1958: "We went smack into next year...snatched the shapes fashion says will dominate '59! Now, here they are...three Coles that're newer-than-new, just when you thought you couldn't find a new [bathing] suit for love or money! Lastex, $25, $22.95, $14.95...Under, Cole's new Power Prifile bra keeps you shapely even while you're wet!"

Collette

Inexpensive clothing. (Example: day dress for $2.99 in 1953.)

Colonial Frocks, Inc.

Expensive clothes. (Example: day dress for about $89.95 in 1950.)

Companion Bags

Bags. (Example: $12.95 in 1955; $13 in 1958.)

Confettis

Shoes. (Example: $16 in 1958.)

Connie

Shoes. (Example: $5.95-$6.95 in 1950.)

Copeland-Patullo (Jo)

Expensive clothes; day dresses beginning at $100.

Cornet

Bags. (Example $10.95 in 1955.)

Crazy Horse

Inexpensive clothes. (Example: day dress for $16 in 1967.)

Crescendoe

Gloves.

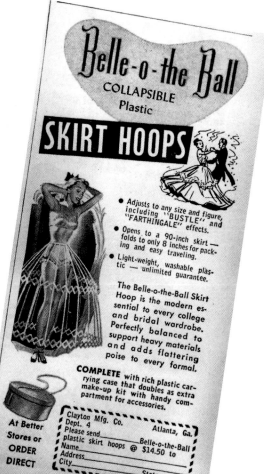

1949

Dale Hilton

Inexpensive clothes. (Example: day dress for $8.95 in 1955.)

Dan Keller

Moderately priced clothes. (Example: day dress for $30 in 1959.)

Dan Millstein

Daryl Creations

Inexpensive clothes. (Example: day dress for about $18 in 1955.)

David Klein

Inexpensive clothing. (Example: evening dress for about $35 in 1957.)

Davids

Inexpensive clothes. (Example: day dress for $6.95 in 1955.)

Dawnelle

Gloves. (Example: $13 in 1958.)

De De Johnson

Moderately priced clothes. (Example: day dress with jacket for $39.95 in 1950.)

DeLiso Debs

Shoes. (Example: $16 in 1950; $18 in 1953.)

Delman

Shoes.

Delmanette

Shoes. (Example: $17 in 1953.)

Dorothy Korby

Inexpensive clothes. (Example: day dress for about $17 in 1958.)

Doris Dodson

Inexpensive clothing. (Example dress for about $15 in 1959.)

Dorset

Inexpensive clothes. (Example: sweater for $6 in 1955.)

Dorshire

Crinolines. (Example: 30 yard crinoline for about $6 in 1957.)

Dress Doctor Co. Inc.

Oscar-winning Hollywood costumer Edith Head was the head of this line. Moderately priced clothes. (Example: day dress for about $55 in 1950.)

Dressner

Bags. (Example: $5 in 1950.)

Dr. Scholl's

Shoes; first found ad in 1959.

Dudley Casuals

Inexpensive clothes. (Example: day dress for $18 in 1955.)

Egret

Hats. (Example: $3.95 in 1955.)

Elfreda-Fox Inc.

Elizabeth Byrne

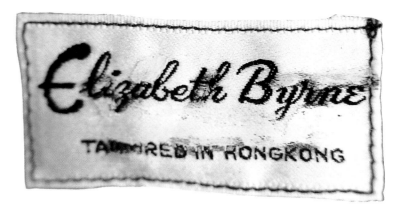

Ellen Brooke

Expensive clothes; dresses began at $100.

Ellen Tracy

Inexpensive clothes. (Example: day dress for $16 in 1967.)

Emma Dombe

Especially popular for her evening wear at moderate prices.

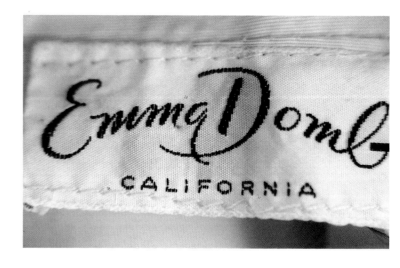

1957

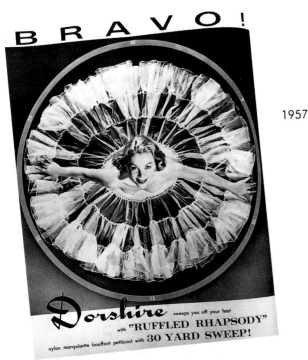

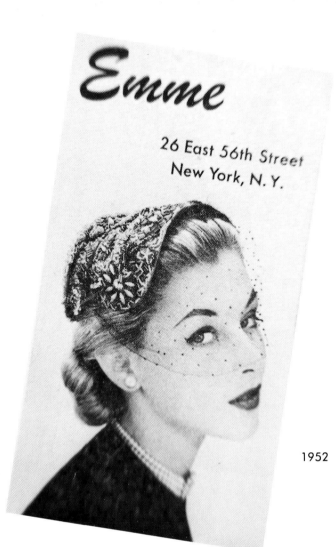

Emme

26 East 56th Street
New York, N.Y.

1952

Emme

    Hats.

Enna Jettick

    Shoes. (Example: $10.95-$12.95 in 1959.)

Everitt

    Hats.

Fiancees

    Shoes. (Example: $13 in 1958.)

Florsheim

    Shoes. (Example: $17 in 1950.)

Foot Flairs

    Shoes. (Example: $11 in 1953.)

Fredrick's of Hollywood

    Ads discovered as early as 1955; 1959 advertisement: "Flaunty Jaunty pullover...clings to your curves dramatically...$4.98; Skanty Dandy permanently pleated flirt skirt...$6.98; Dazzling Dot..sheath [dress] a date-time wonder...$10.95."

Freemold Co.

    Plastic Hoops out of Glen Cove, New York; advertisement in 1955: "Full Skirts Stay Full with Hoop-La. Light as a wisp! Cool as a zephyr! A snap to assemble! Your bouffant and flared skirts will float on air with heavenly "Hoop-La" on the job! Long-lasting, SO comfy! Wear with or without petticoats...You'll look like a fashion model! White only $1.25."

Freshy Playclothes

    Inexpensive clothes. (Example: halter top for about $3, skirt for about $6, shirt for about $4, and shorts for about $3 in 1950.)

Friendly Shoe Co.

    (Example: $7.95 in 1957.)

Fritz Mar

    Inexpsneive clothing. (Example: day dress for about $18 in 1959.)

Gabar

    Bathing suits. (Example: $17 in 1955.)

Gantner of California

    Inexpensive clothing. (Example: playsuit for $17 in 1955.)

Gay Gibson

    Inexpensive clothes. (Example: evening dress for about $20 in 1958; day dress for about $25 in 1960.)

Gene Burton

    Heavily advertised teenager's clothing. (Example: felt circle skirt for $19.95 and jersey blouse for $10.95 in 1956.)

Gertrude Davenport

    Inexpensive clothing. (Example: top for $6.95 in 1955.)

Glenhaven

    Best known for suits; 1955 advertisement: "The suit with the look...casually understated and significantly tailored...to meet the most important people in the most important places!...and the price? Quiet please, it's only $39.95."

Gossard

    Underfashions—especially body shapers; ads found as early as the 1940s.

Gotham

    Stockings.

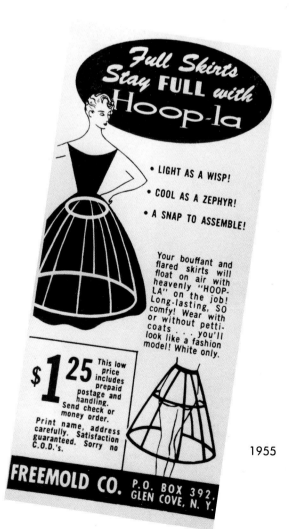

1955

155

Grant Madeleine
  Gloves.
Greta Plattry
  Inexpensive clothes. (Example: shirt for $18 in 1955.)
Handmacher
  Suits; 1955 advertisement: "I have just the man for you...Really, there's nobody like Mr. Handmacher. You never dreamed a suit could fit so flawlessly or look so absolutely right. You can't have him all to yourself, though. He's America's favorite suitmaker." (Example: suit for $79.97 in 1955.)

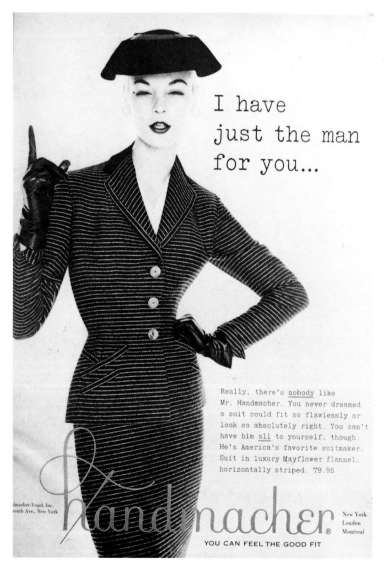

1955

Hanes
  Stockings; first found advertisement in 1955: An illustration of a mermaid with a caption reading "Poor girl! she can't wear seamless stockings by Hanes!" 1957 advertisement: "In 13000 BC smart women wore nothing. In 1957 AD smart women wear nothing but seamless stockings by Hanes." Also in 1957: "Nature gave you seamless legs, Hanes give you seamless stockings. No seams to worry about."

Hannah
  Moderately priced clothes; begun in 1937. (Example: day dress for about $60, and dress suit for $125 in 1955.)
Helen Gudgell
  Moderately price clothes. (Example: day dress for $35 in 1949.)
Henry Bendel
  Moderatelly priced to expensive clothes. (Example: day dress for $35 in 1949; day dress for $175 in 1955.)
Henry Rosenfeld, Inc.
  Inexpensive clothes. (Example: blouse for $3.98, and skirt for $5.98 in 1955; day dress for about $15 in 1958.)
Holeproof Hoisery Co.
  Stockings; first found ad in 1929.
Hollywood-Maxell
  Underfashions, especially bras. (Example: bras $2.50-$5 in 1958.)
Hope Reed
  Inexpensive clothes. (Example: day dress for $10 in 1955.)
House of Lord's
  Moderately priced clothes. (Example: day dress for about $40 in 1955.)
Impressionistic
  Paper clothes.
Irene (of New York)
  Hats.

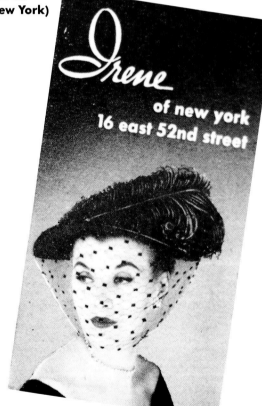

1950

Jack Winter
  "Pants that really fit."
J.B. Martin Shoes
  Shoes.
James Sterling
  Paper clothes.
Jamison
  Moderately priced clothes. (Example: day dress for $55.95 in 1954.)

Jane Holly

Inexpensive clothes. (Example: blouse for about $5 in 1949.)

Jane Irwill

Jane Leslie

Inexpensive clothes. (Example: day dress for $8.99 in 1955.)

Jane Parker

Inexpensive clothes. (Example: day dress for about $25 in 1958.)

Jantsen

Primarily known for bathing suits, but also manufactured—to a limited extent—underfashions; since the 1920s. (Example: bra for $3, sweater for $14.98, and bathing suit for $18.95 in 1957.)

Jay Thorpe

Jerell Juniors

Inexpensive clothing. (Example: day dress for about $25 in 1959.)

Jerry Gideon

Inexpensive clothes. (Example: day dress for about $15 in 1955; day dress for $22.95 in 1958.)

Jerry Greenwald

Moderately priced clothes. (Example: day dress for about $36 in 1955.)

Jesby

Inexpensive fashions. (Example: day dress for $10.95 in 1949.)

Jo Collins

Inexpensive clothes. (Example: day dress for about $15 in 1955; playsuit for about $14, and skirt for about $10 in 1960.)

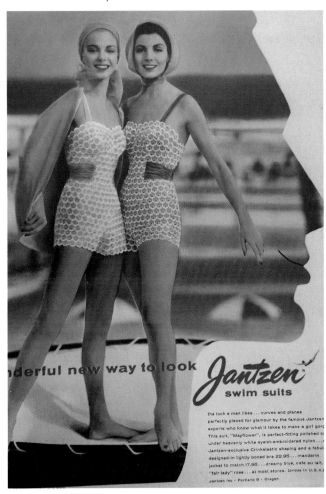

1957

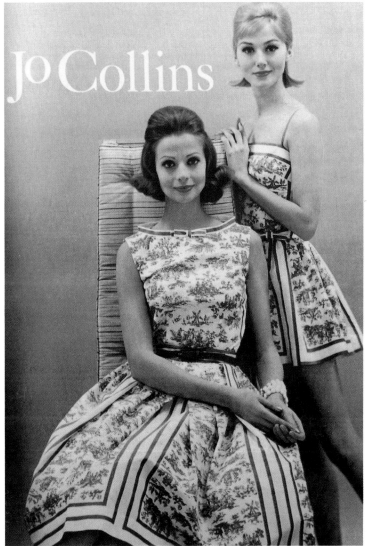

1960

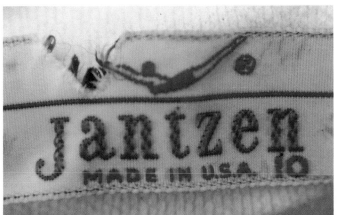

Johansen
   Shoes. (Example: $14 in 1950.)
John Frederico
   Hats. (Example: $12.95 in 1955.)
Jonathan Logan
   Inexpensive clothes. (Example: day dress for about $15 in 1950; dance dress for $17.95 in 1955; day dress for about $18 in 1958; day dress for $14.95 in 1960.)

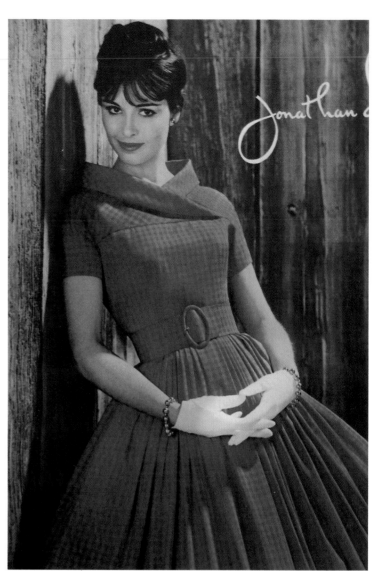

1959

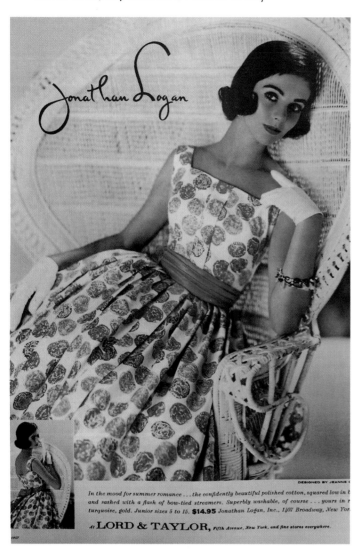

In the mood for summer romance . . . the confidently beautiful polished cotton, squared low in b and sashed with a flash of bow-tied streamers. Superbly washable, of course . . . yours in r turquoise, gold. Junior sizes 5 to 15. **$14.95** *Jonathan Logan, Inc., 1407 Broadway, New Yor*

at **LORD & TAYLOR,** *Fifth Avenue, New York, and fine stores everywhere.*

1957

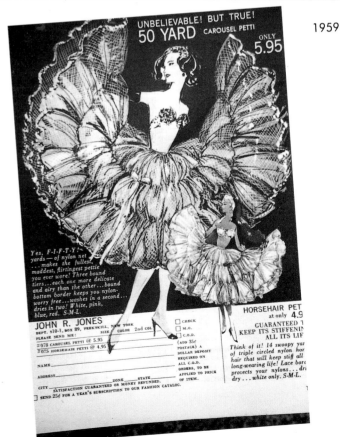

1956

John R. Jones
   Crinolines. Advertisement from 1957: "Unbelievable! But true! 50 yard carousel petti only $5.95. Yes, F-I-F-T-Y! yards— of nylon net...three bound tiers...keeps you nylon worry free!...White, pink, blue, red." (Example: Reversible, two-color crinoline for $3.95, 14 yard horsehair crinoline "guaranteed to keep its stiffening all its life" for $4.95 in 1957.) Advertisement in 1959: "Petti-Pants: [crinoline] petticoat with panties all-in-one. $3.99"

Jordan

Bathing suits; advertisement in 1950: "You'll be a sight for Shore Eyes in this really important new Sea Nymph swim suit by Jordan. The sun-catching fabric is Plisse Lastex...excitingly new and exclusively Sea Nymph. It's dramatically touched with slim-lining ruffles on each side of the front and on the shirred bra; detachable button-on halter strap. Can be worn strapless." About $8.95.

Joselli

Moderately priced clothes. (Example: suit for about $40 in 1949.)

Joseph Guttman

Inexpensive clothes. (Example: day dress for $22.95 in 1955.)

Joset Walker

Moderately priced clothes. (Example: day dress for about $35 in 1953.)

Joyce Hubrite

Inexpensive clothes. (Example: day dress for about $18 in 1955.)

Joy Kingston

Moderately priced clothes. (Example: day dress for $45 in 1949.)

Judy Marshall

Inexpensive clothing. (Example: day dress for $10.95 in 1957.)

Julette Originals

Inexpensive clothes. (Example: day dress for about $25 in 1955.)

Junior Sophisticates

Anne Klein was the head designer for Junior Sophisticates, and actually owned the company. (Example: day dress for $55 in 1955.)

Junior Theme

Inexpensive to moderately priced clothing. (Example: day dress for about $30 in 1959.)

Justin McCarty

Inexpensive clothes. (Example: evening dress for $19.95 in 1949.)

Karen Stark

Expensive clothes. (Example: day dress for $70 in 1955.)

Kathy Karter

Inexpensive clothes. (Example: day dress for $7.98 in 1955.)

Kayser

Stockings and gloves.

Kay Windsor

Inexpensive clothes. (Example: day dress for about $11 in 1955.)

Kelly Arden

Inexpensive clothes. (Example: day dress for $16 in 1967.)

Kenneth Tischler

Moderately priced clothes. (Example: day dress for about $30 in 1953.)

Kislav

Gloves.

Kleinert's

Unusual fashion accessories since the 19th century: ear muffs, bathing caps, corsets, etc. Advertisement in 1957, for a corset-like waist-nipper: "Help yourself to a hand-span waist! Kleinert's 'Waist-In' minimizes your middle like magic! Only $2.98! Don't let your tape measure talk you out of a dream dress...Slip on a Waist-In before you try it on! Its oh-so-strategic boning belittles you, but lets you keep on breathing, too. And Waist-In is made of Feathernap, the textured pure rubber that's feather-soft outside and skin-side. It hooks in front, has adjustable garters..."

Korday

Inexpensive clothes. (Example: playsuit for about $5 in 1950.)

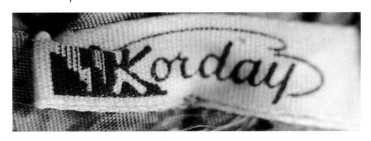

Koret of California

Extremely popular manufacturer of inexpensive clothes. (Example: day dress for $10.95 in 1951; blouse for about $11 in 1958.)

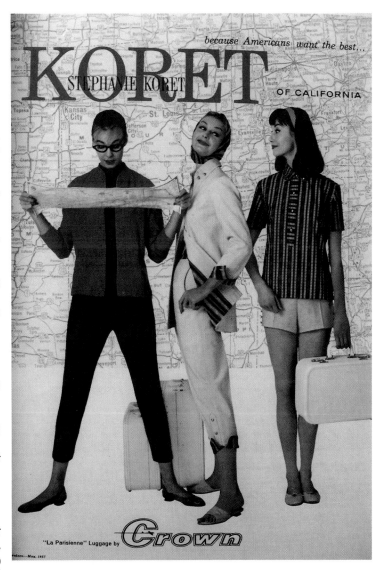

1957

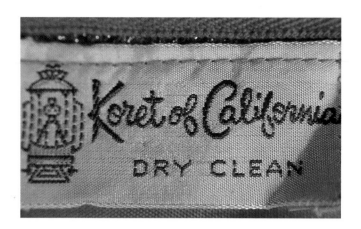

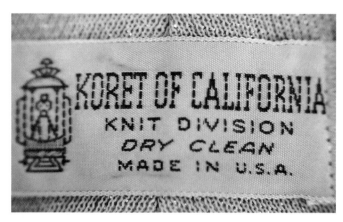

Loomtogs
Inexpensive clothes. (Example: playsuit for $16.95 in 1959.)

Lorrie Deb
Inexpensive "Important Occasion Dresses" for teen-agers. (Example: day dress for $28 in 1957.)

Lotte of Drewyn
Inexpensive clothes. (Example: day dress for about $25 in 1953.)

Louis Gerst
Suits. (Example: $50-$65 in 1949.)

Lov-é
Bras from about the 1940s forward.

L.S. Ayres & Co.

Luxite
Stockings.

Madcaps
Hats.

Mademoiselle
Shoes. (Example: $13 in 1950.)

Krippendorf
Shoes.

Lana Lobell
Inexpensive clothing, particularly popular among young women. (Example: day dress for $10.95 in 1957; day dress for $6.95 in 1959.)

Lanz Originals
Inexpensive to moderately priced clothes. (Example: day dress for about $25 in 1955; day dress for $30 in 1958.)

Larry Aldrich

Laura Mae Life
Inexpensive clothes; advertisement in 1950: "Blouse washes like a Hanky! At good stores everywhere. $2.95." (Example: blouse for $6.99 in 1959.)

Leonard Arkin
Moderately priced clothes. (Example: day dress for about $75 in 1958.)

Leslie Fay
Inexpensive clothes. (Example: day dress for about $23 in 1955; day dress for about $25 in 1958.)

Leslie Morris

Leslie Roberts
Inexpensive clothes. (Example: blouse & skirt for about $8 each, and dress for about $15 in 1950.)

Lewella
Underfashions; 1955 advertisement: "Just picture yourself in 3-D wearing a Lewella convertible sports bra!"

Lilli Ann

Lilly Daché
Lilly Daché was especially known for her hats, but she also had a couture line of dresses, etcetera.

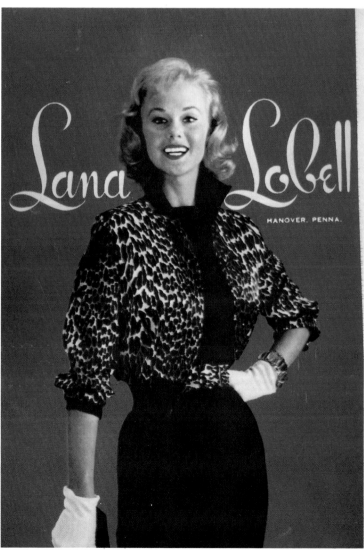

1957

Maidenform

One of the first manufacturers of bras (beginning in the 1930s); their "I dreamed..." ad campaign was legendary...1949: "I dreamed I went to a carnival in my Maidenform bra"; 1952: "I dreamed I was bewitching in my Maidenform bra"; 1959: "I dreamed I was a medieval maiden in my Maidenform bra"; and, in Seventeen magazine, 1959: "I dreamed I was tied to the telephone 25 hours a day in my Maidenform bra." (Example: $1.75 in 1950.)

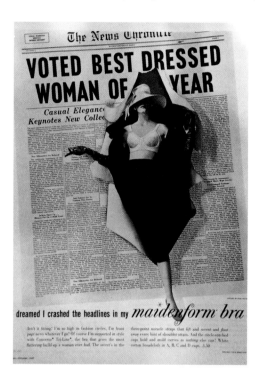

1957

Majestic Specialties

Inexpensive clothes. (Example: day dress for about $11 in 1950.)

Mallory

Hats.

Mam'selle

Bags. (Example: $11 in 1958.)

Mandels of California

Shoes. (Example: $14.98 in 1953; $8.98 in 1955.)

Mannings

Stockings.

Marcel Wagner

Gloves. (Example: $4 in 1958.)

Marquise

Shoes.

Mars Manufacturing ("Mars of Asheville")

Best known for their paper clothes of the late 1960s; before this time, the company manufactured stockings.

Martinique

Shoes.

Mary Allen

Inexpensive clothes. (Example: day dress for $12.98 in 1950.)

Mason

Shoes.

Matty Talmack, Inc.

Expensive clothes; since 1950, dresses beginning at $200.

Max Mayer's

Gloves.

McKettrick

Inexpensive clothes. (Example: day dress for $11 in 1955; day dress for about $13, and day dress about $23 in 1958.)

Mel-Ton

Bags. (Example: $12.95 in 1955.)

Mildred Orrick

Mode O'Day Corp.

Inexpensive clothes. (Example: "House Frock" for $2.99 in 1950.)

Modern Juniors

Inexpensive clothing. (Example: skirt with attached crinoline for $14.95 in 1957.)

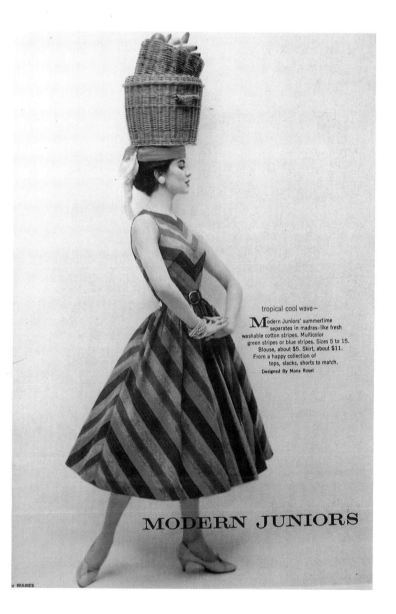

tropical cool wave—

Modern Juniors' summertime separates in madras-like fresh washable cotton stripes. Multicolor green stripes or blue stripes. Sizes 5 to 15. Blouse, about $5. Skirt, about $11. From a happy collection of tops, slacks, shorts to match. Designed By Mona Roset

MODERN JUNIORS

1958

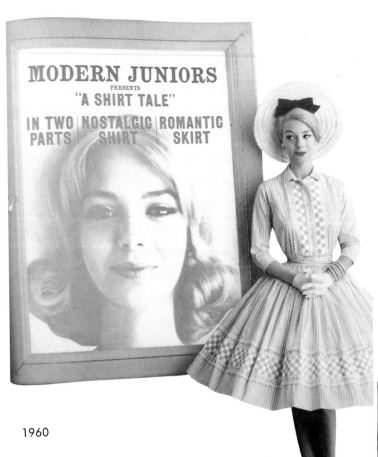

1960

Mojud
 Stockings.
Mollie Parnis
 Expensive clothes; day dresses beginning at $150.
Mort Schrader
 Inexpensive to moderately priced clothes. (Example: evening dress for about $60 in 1958.)
Mr. Alf
 Hats.
Munsingwear
 Stockings.
Murray Goldstein
 Inexpensive clothes. (Example: day dress for $22.95 in 1949.)
Murray Nieman
 Inexpensive clothes. (Example: dress ensemble for $50 in 1955.)
Nadine Formals
 Primarily prom and other teen-age formals; still creates teen formals today. (Example: prom dress for about $30 in 1957.)
Natalie Berne
 Inexpensive to moderately priced clothes. (Example: suit for $35 in 1949.)
Nat Kaplan
Nelly de Grab
 Inexpensive clothes. (Example: blouse for $11 in 1950.)

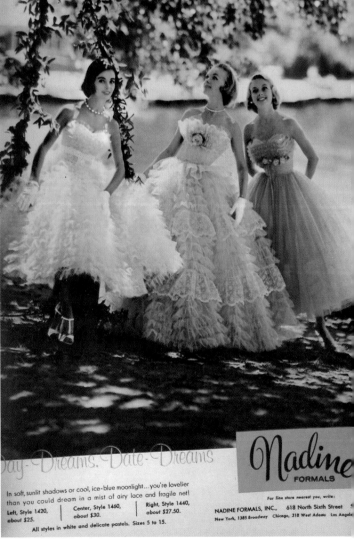

Day-Dreams, Date-Dreams

Nadine
FORMALS

In soft, sunlit shadows or cool, ice-blue moonlight...you're lovelier than you could dream in a mist of airy lace and fragile net!
Left, Style 1420, about $25. | Center, Style 1460, about $30. | Right, Style 1440, about $27.50.
All styles in white and delicate pastels. Sizes 5 to 15.

For fine store nearest you, write:
NADINE FORMALS, INC.   618 North Sixth Street
New York, 1385 Broadway Chicago, 318 West Adams Los Angeles

1957

Nelly Don
Inexpensive to moderately priced clothes. (Example: day dress for $11, suit for $30, and day dress for $30 in 1955.)

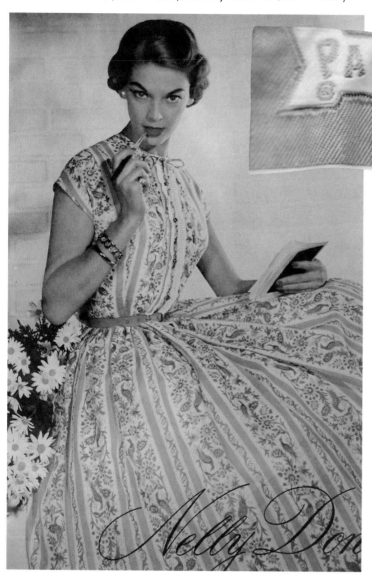

1955

Nettie Rosenstein
Newton Elkin
Shoes.
Nina
Inexpensive clothing. (Example: bathing suit for $25 in 1957.)
No Mend
Stockings.
Olga
Bodyshapers and corsetry. (Example: corset for $16.50 in 1955.)
Palmdayl
Inexpensive clothes. (Example: slacks for $4 in 1955.)
Palter DeLiso (see also DeLiso)
Shoes.
Pandora Footwear
Shoes.

Pantsville
Women's pants.

Paraphernalia
Best known for wacky 1960s clothing, including paper dresses; their vinyl "Glue It Yourself" dress sold for $15 + $5 for foil scraps, stars, etcetera so owner could decorate as pleased; Betsey Johnson of Paraphernalia described the company's philosophy; she said they loved fabrics "you'd spray with Windex, rather than dryclean...We were into plastic flash synthetics that looked like synthetics. It was: 'Hey, your dress looks like my shower curtain!'"
Paris Shop
Inexpensive clothes; advertisement in 1959: "Zip-Off...$8.95...It pleases you because the cleverly concealed waistline zipper whisks the skirt off in a jiffy, revealing a stunning sheath dress." (Example: blouse for $2.99 in 1951; day dress for $6.99, and blouse for $2.99 in 1955; day dress for $5.99 in 1959.)

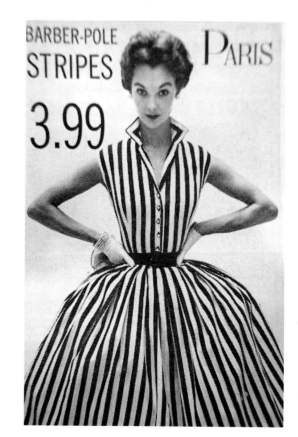

1955

163

Par-Form
   Bathing suits. (Example: about $13 in 1950.)
Patricia Fiar
   Inexpensive clothes. (Example: day dress for $17.95 in 1955.)
Peck & Peck (Tweeds of Scotland)
Peg Palmer
   Inexpensive clothes. (Example: day dress for about $18 in 1952.)
Penn Delphia Shoes
   Shoes.
Peter Pan
   Underfashions. (Example: bras for $1.50-$5 in 1949; "New Basque Slip...All-in-one: Slip, torso slimmer, and bra" $14.95 in 1955.)
Petti
   Inexpensive clothes. (Example: skirt for about $17 in 1960; day dress for $19 in 1967.)
Philoppe Tournay
Phoenix
   Stockings.
Pierre
   Shoes.
Playtex
   Bodyshapers; 1949 advertisement for a panty girdle: "Mildred O'Donnell, famous diving and swimming champion: 'Playtex is invisible under all clothes, from bathing suits to new summer fashions!'" $3.50; 1955 advertisement: "Invisible under the sleekest [bathing] suit, a latex panty girdle shaped to smooth the way for a closely figured swimsuit..." $5.
Prim Fashion
   Inexpensive clothes. (Example: day dress for about $23 in 1952.)
Mary Quant
   A popular 1960s fashion designer who plugged the mini skirt; she designed not only on her own, but also with other manufacturers, including J.C. Penny. Her clothes were noted for being affordable and hip.
QualiCraft
   Shoes. (Example: $5.99 in 1950.)
R & K Originals·
   Inexpensive clothes. (Example: day dress for about $20 in 1958.)
Red Cross Shoes
   Shoes.
Reel Poise
   Bathing suits. (Example: $17 in 1955.)
Reid & Reid
   Inexpensive clothes. (Example: day dress for about $15 in 1950.)
Rembrant
   Moderately priced clothes. (Example: day dress for $60 in 1959.)
Richard Cole
   Moderately priced clothes. (Example: day dress for about $60 in 1958.)
Roger Van S.
   Bags.
Rose Marie Reid
   Inexpensive clothes. (Example: bathing suit for $11 in 1955.)

Russ Togs
   Inexpensive clothing. (Example: day dress for about $11, and blouse for under $5 in 1959.)
Sacony
   Inexpensive clothes. (Example: day dress for $14.95 in 1950; skirt for $8.98, blouse for $2.98, and shorts for $3.98 in 1956.)
Saks Shoes
   1958 advertisement: "Serving the nation for 26 years." (Example: $4.99 in 1958.)
Sally V
   Hats.
Sanson
   Stockings.
Scott Paper Products
   Paper clothes.
Screen Styles
   Inexpensive clothes. (Example: "Tel-A-Vision Blouse" for $5.95 in 1950.)
Selby Shoes
   Fashion shoes designed for good health, with supportive arches.
Seymour Jacobson
   Moderate to expensive clothes. (Example: evening dress for about $110 in 1952.)
Shalimar
   Gloves.
Sheila Lynn
Shelton Stroller
   Inexpensive clothes. (Example: day dress for $8.95 in 1951; day dress for $13 in 1955.)
Shenanigans
   Shoes. (Example: $14.95-$15.95 in 1950.)
Shirely Lee
   Inexpensive clothing. (Example: day dress for about $15 in 1957.)

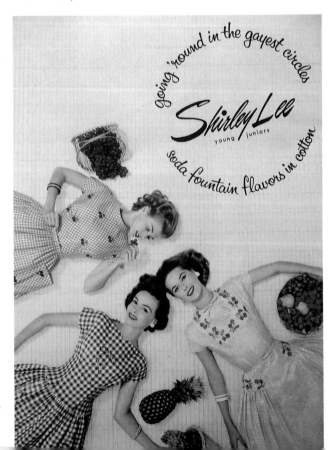

going 'round in the gayest circles
Shirley Lee
young juniors
soda fountain flavors in cotton

1958

Sidran of Dallas
  Inexpensive clothes. (Example: day dress for $29.95 in 1955.)

Signature
  Stockings.

Simmon Co.
  Paper clothes.

Skippies
  Bodyshapers. (Example: $3.95-$10.95 in 1953.)

Sloat & Co.
  Inexpensive clothes.

Solby Bayers
  Shoes (Example: $12.95 in 1953.)

Sportsmasters of California
  Sportsclothes. (Example: bathing suit for about $14 in 1958.)

Stephanie Koret
  Inexpensive clothes. (Example: skirt for $7.95, and jacket for $8.95 in 1949.)

Stephanie
  Moderately priced clothes. (Example: day dress for about $30 in 1955.)

Strutwear
  Stockings, lingerie, and blouses; 1958 advertisement: "Strutwear nylons with provocative dark seams. In glamorous fashion-tested shades."

Sue Brett
  Inexpensive clothes. (Example: jumper for about $23 in 1958.)

Superb
  Gloves.

Surf Togs
  Bathing Suits. (Example: $12.98 in 1957.)

Susan Todd
  Moderately priced clothes. (Example: day dress for about $35 in 1959.)

Susan Thomas
  Inexpensive clothes. (Example: blouse for about $11, and blouse for about $8 in 1951; day dress for $15 in 1955.)

Tall-Girl
  Tall Girl began advertising in the last few years of the 1940s, and continued to grow in popularity throughout the 1960s. As their name suggests, they specialized in fashions for taller women.

Teena Paige
  Inexpensive clothing, particularly popular among young women. (Example: day dress for about $23 in 1957; day dress for about $15 in 1960.)

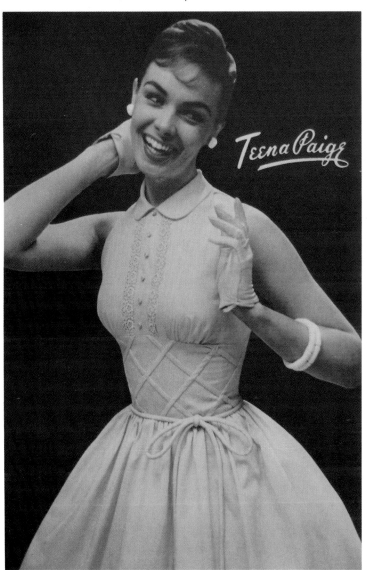

1957

Tiger Tissue
  Paper clothes.

Toni Edwards
  Inexpensive to moderately priced clothing. (Example, day dress for about $30 in 1957.)

Toni Owen
  Inexpensive clothes. (Example: blouse for $14.95 and skirt for $8.95 in 1949.)

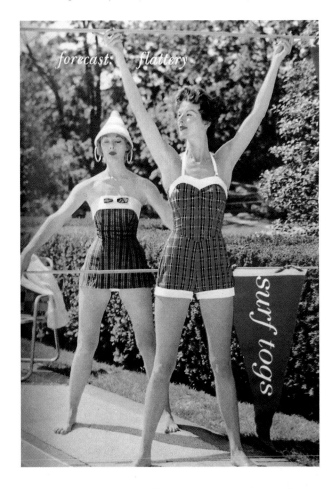

1957

Townfield

Inexpensive clothes. (Example: day dress for about $23 in 1958.)

Town Tailored

Inexpensive clothes. (Example: day dress for about $20 in 1955.)

Treadeasy

Shoes. (Example: $12.95-$14.95 in 1952.)

Treo

Bodyshapers, since the 1920s.

Trudy Hall

Inexpsensive clothing. (Example: day dress for $10.95 in 1957.)

Turner Togs

Casual wear. (Example: pants for about $4 in 1957.)

Tuscancy

Paper clothes.

Tweedie

Shoes.

Valentine Shoe Co.

Valerie Modes

Hats.

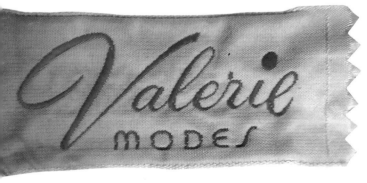

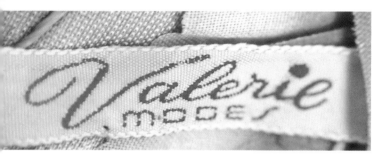

Vallejo Gantner

Van Raalte

Gloves, stockings (including seamless), and underfashions; a 1955 advertisement pushed faux doeskin gloves.

Vera Maxwell

Moderately priced to expensive clothes, since 1952; sold to about 300 stores; suits began at $150.

Vicky Vaughn

Inexpensive clothing. Slogan: "Only the look is expensive." (Example, day dress for $14.95 in 1957; day dress for about $10 in 1960.)

Vision

Shoes.

Vitality

Shoes.

Walter Katten

Specialized in fur bags.

Warner's

Underfashions. (Example: bra for $1, and girdle for $3.50 in 1949; bra for $2.50 in 1959.)

Weber Originals

Inexpensive clothes. (Example: blouse for $4 in 1955.)

Wesley Simpson

Inexpensive clothes. (Example: day dress for about $25 in 1950.)

Westover

Inexpensive clothes. (Example: day dress for about $11 in 1950.)

Whiting & Davis

Since the late 19th century, famous for bags made of metal mesh; since the 1930s, also made—to a lesser extent—metal mesh belts and other accessories.

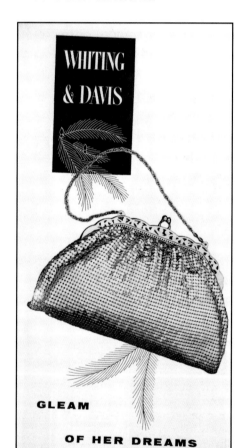

1955

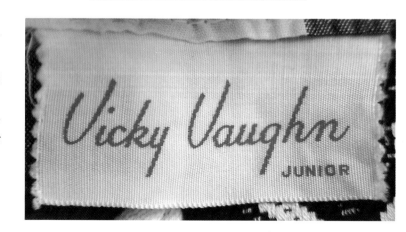

Wilco Fashions
 Inexpensive clothes. (Example: playsuit for $4.95 in 1955.)

Will Steinman
 Moderately priced to expensive clothes. (Example: evening dress for $110 in 1955.)

Wohl Shoe Co.

Wyner

Young Edwardians
 Best known for their Victorian-inspired "granny" type clothes of the late 1960s and 1970s, but also produced other types of women's clothing.

Youth Guild (see also Anne Fogarty)
 Inexpensive clothes. (Example: day dress for $25 in 1955.)

The average woman could not afford traditional couture garments—whether custom or ready-to-wear. It is a rarity for collectors today to discover a couture original (that is, a garment custom made for a client); however, ready-to-wear couture garments are more accessible. This list points out the most prominent designers of the 1950s and 60s—those who had either custom houses and/or ready-to-wear lines which they owned or which carried their own labels. Often coutures worked under other coutures before they went off on their own, but this work was often anonymous, and is not noted here. Whenever possible, notes have been given if the couture was a specialist, when they had their first line, and when their house closed.

Adolfo
 Hats; originally worked for Bergdorf Goodman, but in 1962, went out on his own; soon after, he had a ready-to-wear clothing line, in addition to hats.

Hardy Amies
 Opened in 1945; had both a custom and ready-to-wear business.

Cristobal Balenciaga
 Opened in the 1930s; retired in 1968.

Pierre Balmain
 Opened 1945; in 1951, began a ready-to-wear line.

Geoffrey Beane
 Opened a couture ready-to-wear line in 1963; his less expensive line is "Beane Bag."

Pierre Cardin
 Started his first women's line in 1957; his first women's ready-to wear line began six years later.

Hattie Carnegie
 Opened in 1918; Carnegie died in 1956, and her house discontinued soon after.

Bonnie Cashin
 Opened in 1954.

Oleg Cassini
 In 1961, Cassini was appointed Jacqueline Kennedy's official designer.

John Cavanagh
 Opened in 1952; began his ready-to-wear line in the 1960s.

Gabrielle (Coco) Chanel
 Opened 1912; closed 1939; reopened in 1954.

Clive
 Opened in 1961 with custom and ready-to-wear lines.

Lilly Daché
 Hats; also clothing; Dache's first hats were created c.1924; her first clothing line appeared in 1949.

Oscar de la Renta
 Opened his own house in 1965.

Christian Dior
 First line appeared in 1947; Dior died in 1957, but his house continued.

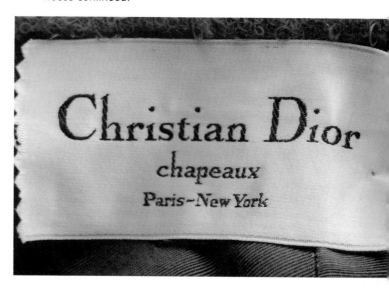

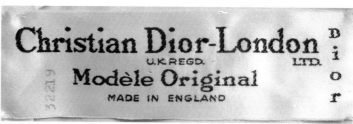

Jaques Fath
 Opened 1937; first ready-to-wear line in 1948.

Hubert Givenchy
 Opened in 1952.

Alix Grés
 From 1934, was known by his full name; his house closed during WWII, but reopened after the war under the name "Grés."

Jacques Heim
 Sportswear; opened in 1930s; closed 1966.

Hermés
 Hermés gloves and bags date from 1837; by the 1960s, they were also well known for their scarves.

Anne Klein
 Opened in 1968; previously designed and owned Junior Sophisticates (see mass-manufacturer's list).

Guy Laroche
 Opened in 1957; ready-to-wear line appeared in 1960.

Mainbocher
 Opened in 1930; closed in 1971.

Claire McCardell
 First label appeared in 1941.

Edward Molyneaux

Opened in 1919. In 1950, Molyneaux closed all but one of his houses and retired; 15 years later, he tried to make a comeback with a ready-to-wear line, but it was unsuccessful and he retired again shortly after.

Jean Muir

Opened in 1961 under the name Jane & Jane; in 1966, Muir opened her own company and began using her full name.

Norman Norell

Opened his own house in 1960.

Lilly Pulitzer

Opened in 1958; closed in 1984.

Yves Saint Laurent

Took over Dior's house after his death; opened his own house in 1962; in 1966 began a ready-to-wear line.

Elsa Schiaparelli

Opened in 1929; closed in 1954.

Victor Stiebel

Opened in 1932; closed during WWII, but reopened shortly after the war.

Sally Victor

Hats; millinery from her premiere collection could cost some $1,000 for hats including fur and jewels; her ready-to-wear line was sold under the name "Sally V"; she opened in 1934 and retired in 1968.

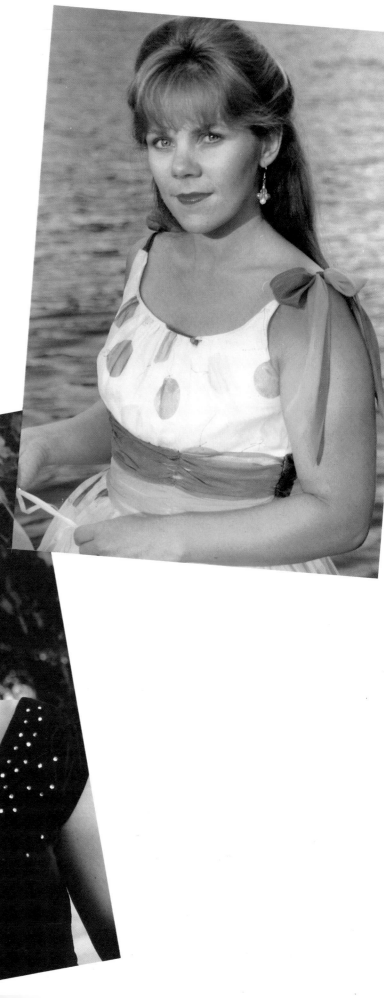

Selected Bibliography

Primary Sources—Periodicals

American Girl
Charm
Glamour
Good Housekeeping
Harper's Bazaar
Ladies' Home Journal
Mademoiselle
McCall's Pattern Fashions
Montgomery Ward Catalog
Seventeen
Today's Woman
Vogue
Women's Wear Daily

Primary Sources—Books

Daves, Jessica. *Ready-To-Wear Miracle*. G.P. Putnam's Sons: New York, 1967.
Post, Emily. *Emily Post's Etiquette*. Funk & Wagnalls: New York 1965-69.
Rathbone, Lucy and Elizabeth Tarpley. *Fabrics & Dress*. Houghton Mifflin Co.: Cambridge, Mass., 1948.

Secondary Sources—Periodicals

Brightman, Joan. "Paper Power: The Sixties Paper Clothing Phenomenon." *Vintage Fashions*, Hobby House Press, Inc.: Cumberland, MD, January 1992.

Secondary Sources—Books

Charles-Roux, Edmonde. *Chanel & Her World*. Vendome Press: London, 1981.
Ewing, Elizabeth. *Dress and Undress*. B.T. Batsford, Ltd.: London, 1978.
Ginsburg, Madeleine, Avril Hart, and Valerie D. Mendes. *Four Hundred Years of Fashion*. Victoria And Albert Museum: London, 1984.

Keenan, Brigette. *Dior In Vogue*. Octopus: London, 1981.
Kennett, Frances. *Collector's Book of Twentieth Century Fashion*. Granada: London, 1983.
Lencek, Lena and Gideon Bosker. *Making Waves*. Chronicle Books: San Francisco, 1989.
Lobenthal, Joel. *Radical Rags*. Abbeville Press: New York, 1990.
O'Hara, Georgina. *The Encyclopaedia of Fashion*. Harry N. Abrams, Inc.: New York, 1986.
Shaeffer, Claire B. *Couture Sewing Techniques*. Taunton Press, Inc.: Newton, CT, 1994.
Shields, Jody. *Hats: A Stylish History*. Clarkson Potter: NY, 1991.
Yarwood, Doreen. *The Encyclopedia of Costume*. Bonanza Books: NY, 1978.

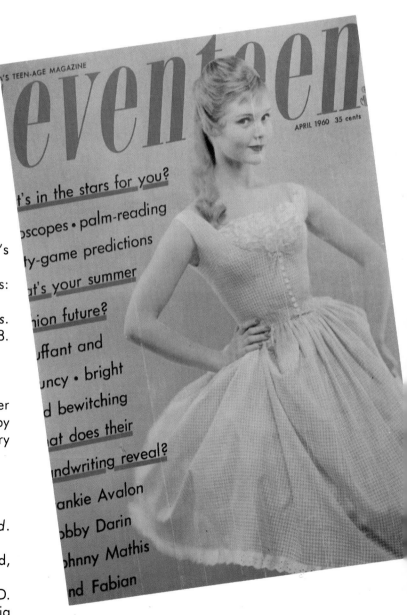

Value Guide

The following is only intended as a guide for collectors and dealers who want to know the general sale prices for collectible fashions from the 1950s forward. The listed prices come directly from dealers throughout the United States, and reflect items in excellent to mint condition. Bear in mind that sale prices vary from state to state, and from region to region; demand in your own area and current collecting trends also affect values.

When evaluating items, every bit of damage and every flaw must be taken into consideration, and the items must be depreciated accordingly. Because fashions from the 1950s forward are still quite plentiful, any items not in excellent condition have very low values, or no collecting value at all.

Page	Item	Value	Page	Item	Value
1, 84	Hat	$50–60	33	Dress	$20–30
1, 38	Dress	$25–40	24	Bodice & Skirt	$25–40
3, 98, 99	Dress	$30–40	24, 25	Dresses	$25–45 each
3, 62	Bathing Suit & Jacket	$25–40	36	Dress	$10–25
4, 114	Dior Dress	$40–50	36, 37	Skirt	$10–25
5, 7, 49	Dress	$20–30	37	Dress	$15–25
6, 106	Dress	$25–35	38, 39	Chinese Dress	$40–70
6, 136	Hat	$25–30	39	Dombe Dress	$45–75
6, 119	Dress	$35–65	40, 41	Simpson Dress	$35–65
7, 50, 51	Varsity Jacket	$25–30	41	Lace Dress	$40–65
7, 116	Dress	$25–35	43	2–piece Dress	$20–30
7, 69	Bathing Suit	$15–25	43	House Dress	$20–30
8, 20	Dress	$75–85	44	Dress	$25–45
8, 52, 53	Dress	$25–35	45	Skirt	$15–30
8, 86	Dress	$35–45	46	Dress & Sweater	$25–40
10, 11	Suit	$50–65	46, 47	Striped Dress	$30–40
13, 168	Dress	$35–50	47	Cotton Dress	$10–15
14	Dress	$40–60	47	Lace Dress	$30–45
15	Dress	$20–35	48	Dombe Dress	$95–120
16	Dress	$10–30	48	Suit–Dress	$20–30
17	Dress	$35–50	49	Suit	$50–70
18	Skirt	$30–45	50	Suit	$20–30
21	Dress	$20–30	50, 51	Skirt	$50–65
22	Dress	$50–60	53	Skirt	$20–35
23	Dress	$25–50	53	Blouse	$10–15
24	Skirt	$10–20	54	Dress	$30–40
25	Dress	$25–35	55	Dresses	$25–35 each
26	Skirt	$10–20	56	Poodle Skirt	$70–100
26	Blouse	$10–15	56	Dress	$10–20
30	Bridal Gown	$50–75	57	Skirt	$30–50
31	Bridal Gown	$100–150	58	Dress	$20–30
31	Headdress	$10–15	59, 168	Dress	$40–65
32	Pattern	$5–10	60	Play Suit	$35–45
32, 33	2–piece Dress	$20–30	61	Sweater	$45–65

Page	Item	Value
125	Pants	$10–25 each
126	Ponytail Bathing Cap	$10–15
126	Hair Bathing Caps	$10–15 each
126	Olympic Bathing Cap	$5–10
127	Purse	$3–10
127	Hat	$5–15
127	Green Hat	$5–10
128	Dior Hats	$25–35 each
129	Stockings in Packaging	$25–30
129	Hat	$3–10
130	Purse	$3–10
130	Pillbox Hat	$5–10
130	Burgundy Hat	$15–25
131	Hats	$3–10 each
131	Stockings in Box	$5–15
132	Purse	$3–10
132	Bow Hat	$15–20
132	Pillbox Hat	$3–10
133	Hat	$5–20
134	Feather Hat	$15–25
134, 135	Velvet Hat	$30–45
135	Shoes	$20–25
136	Feather Hats	$30–50 each
137	Purse	$3–10
137	Dior Hat	$30–45
138	Miss Paper Dress	$20–35
138	Yellow Pages Dress	$20–30
139	Dress	$25–35
140	Dress in Packaging	$30–40
140	Dress	$20–30
141	Dress	$10–20
142	Dress	$5–10
143	Dress	$5–10
144	Dress	$20–40
145	Suit	$10–25
145	Dress	$20–30
146	Dress	$30–40
152	Magazine	$10–25
169	Magazine	$10–15

Page	Item	Value	Page	Item	Value
61	Pants	$30–40	91	Dress	$20–30
63	Sunglasses	$30–45	92	Dress	$25–35
63	Sweater	$30–45	93	Dress	$25–35
64	3–piece Play Suit	$20–25	94	Dress	$10–25
64	Bathing Cap	$10–15	95	Skirt	$20–25
65	Halter Top	$10–20	95	Dress	$15–20
65	Bathing Suit	$15–20	96	Ribbon Dress	$40–65
66	Top	$10–15	96	Crochet Dress	$25–35
67	Pants	$15–25	96, 97	Bubble Dress	$50–75
67	Belt	$3–5	97	Chinese Ensemble	$30–45
68	Play Suit	$15–20	98	Striped Dress	$20–25
68	Sweater	$30–40	99	Lace Dress	$10–25
69	Bathing Suits	$15–25 each	100	Chiffon Dress	$15–30
70	Play Suit	$10–15	100, 101	2–piece Dress	$35–60
70	Pants	$30–45	101	Taffeta Dress	$20–30
72	Hat	$5–10	102	Ensemble	$45–75
72	Shoes	$25–35	103	Ribbon Ensemble	$40–65
73	Hat	$25–35	103	Dress	$25–35
74	Purse	$10–20	104	Pantsuit	$40–65
74	Shoes	$25–40	105	Dress	$40–70
74	Hat	$15–25	106	Beaded Dress	$80–120
75	Clutch	$15–25	106	Knit Dress	$25–40
75	Bag	$20–30	107	Lace Dress	$25–35
75	Shoes	$25–35	107	Trapeze Dress	$25–35
75	Hat	$5–10	108	Knit Dress	$20–30
76	Purse	$10–15	108	Lace Dress	$20–30
76	Hat	$25–35	109	Suit–Dress	$15–25
77	Armadillo Bag	$65–75	109	Knit Outfit	$20–40
77	Purse	$30–35	109	Silk Dress	$35–50
77	Shoes	$15–25	110	Suit	$30–45
78	Hats	$10–20 each	111	Polyester Dress	$10–20
78	Shoes in Box	$25–40	111	Metallic Dress	$30–45
79	Ostrich Hat	$55–65	112	Dress	$25–35
79	Skeleton Hat	$15–25	113	Trained Dress	$10–25
79	Valerie Modes Hat	$10–20	113	2–piece Dress	$30–40
80	Stockings in Box	$15–25 each	115	Chiffon Dress	$10–25
80	Hat	$5–10	115	Chinese Dress	$20–30
80	Shoes	$25–30	116	Suit	$25–40
81	Plume Hat	$25–35	117	Dress	$20–35
81	Straw Hat	$5–10	117	Bridal Gown	$25–40
81	Satin Hat	$30–40	118	Beaded Bridal Dress	$70–100
82	Marabou Hat	$35–50	118	Tucked Bridal Dress	$75–100
82	Beak Hat	$25–40	119	Nautical Dress	$10–25
82	Purse	$15–20	120, 148	Girl Scout Uniform	$30–40
82	Shoes	$20–30	120, 121	Knit Ensemble	$20–25
83	Bag	$10–25	121	Dress	$20–30
83	Shoes	$20–40	122	Beaded Dress	$75–100
83	Hat	$5–10	122	Knit Dress	$25–30
84	Shoes	$25–35	123	Dress	$20–30
85	Ensemble	$25–40	123	Lei	$3–5
87	Dress	$25–35	124	J.F.K. Dress	$85–$125
89	Dress	$25–30	124	T–shirt	$10–20
90	Dress	$35–50	124	Pants	$10–25

Modeling Credits

Anna Kristine Crivello: 46 56 (R), 63 (TR), 91, 120 (T & M), 148.

Clinton McKay Crivello: 7, 50, 51, 58.

Lisa Ann Crivello: 3 (BL), 5, 6 (T), 8 (B), 13, 21, 38 (T), 39 (M), 49 (M), 50 (T), 51 (M), 55, 58, 59, 62, 63 (TL), 86, 87, 92, 98 (B), 100 (T & BL), 104, 106 (M & B), 110, 111 (TL & BL), 113 (T & BL), 115 (T), 116 (B), 119 (T), 122 (TR), 123, 124 (M), 146, 168.

Lisa Dunn: 94.

Joslin Gordon: 6 (T), 23, 35 (TL & B), 40, 41 (L), 101 (TR & B), 113 (BR), 115 (B), 122 (TL & B), 143.

Darcie Jones:1 (TL), 3 (BR), 4, 8 (T), 15, 20, 24, 30, 32, 33 (B), 34 (L), 39 (R), 43 (T & M), 45, 48, 50 (BL), 54, 57, 60, 64 (TR), 65 (BL), 66, 67, 68 (B), 69 (T & BL), 70, 72, 75, 79 (T), 84, 90, 95 (T), 96 (TL), 98 (T), 99 (T), 100 (BR), 101 (TL), 103 (TR & B), 107 (B), 109 (T), 111 (TR & BR), 112, 114, 116 (T), 118 (TL), 124 (B), 125, 126 (MR), 137, 138 (T), 139, 145 (T & M).

Stephanie Jones: 1 (TR), 6 (B), 8 (M), 16, 22, 31, 34 (R), 35 (TR), 37, 38 (B), 41 (R), 47 (B), 52, 53 (B), 65 (TR & BR), 69 (M & BR), 73, 74, 76, 78 (L), 79 (B), 81 (BL), 82, 85, 93, 96 (TR), 97 (T & BR), 99 (M & B), 103 (TL), 105, 106 (TL), 107 (T), 108 (B), 109 (BL), 117, 119 (B), 121 (T & M), 126 (T, ML, & B), 127, 128, 129, 130, 131, 132, 133, 134 (T), 136, 138 (B), 142, 144, 145 (B).

Jennifer Yarascak: 10, 11, 14, 17, 18, 25, 26, 33 (T), 36, 43 (B), 44, 47 (T), 49 (T & BL), 53 (T), 56 (L), 61, 64 (TL), 68 (T), 78 (R), 80, 81 (T & BR), 83, 89, 95 (B), 96 (B), 97 (BL), 102, 108 (T), 109 (BR), 118 (TR & B), 120 (B), 121 (BL), 124 (T), 134 (B), 135, 140, 141.

Index

SEP 18 1997